Do Not Forsake Me

Do Not Forsake Me

Support for Dementia Caregivers

PAUL RADER

WIPF & STOCK · Eugene, Oregon

DO NOT FORSAKE ME
Support for Dementia Caregivers

Wipf & Stock
An Imprint of Wipf and Stock Publishers
199 W. 8th Ave., Suite 3
Eugene, OR 97401

www.wipfandstock.com

PAPERBACK ISBN: 979-8-3852-2272-8
HARDCOVER ISBN: 979-8-3852-2273-5
EBOOK ISBN: 979-8-3852-2274-2

VERSION NUMBER 08/28/24

The author wishes to acknowledge grant support from the Louisville Institute.

To Ava, Allie,
Brooks, Lochlan,
& Fritz

Do not cast me away when I am old;
Do not forsake me when my strength is gone.

—Ps 71:9

Contents

Introduction

As word got out that I would be writing a book on caring for those with dementia, I began to receive comments, articles and information from friends and acquaintances—letters, emails, messages of all sorts. Some told me jokes about it. (Did you hear about the old friends who are now new friends?) Most of all, people told me their stories. Stories about someone they know (or knew). Stories about their mother or father or grandparents. They told me about their fears for themselves.

For example, I sat beside a woman from Nebraska on a flight from Atlanta to Paris who told me about her mother, who had had Alzheimer's disease for nearly ten years before dying at the age of eighty-three. I was told her mother lived at home for most of those years, was taken care of by her husband, and was "really no trouble at all" (most of the time) except that she would get out of the house and wander off. Two sets of locks were installed on the doors and windows, yet she would still occasionally manage to escape. "She was like Houdini." I was told her final illness lasted but a few weeks, and that the family was grateful it hadn't been worse.

It seems that we in the church—and in America at large—are finally waking up to just how pervasive a condition dementia is. The Presbyterian Older Adult Ministries Network at its annual conference last year (September 14–15, 2023) included a presentation on "What Should I Know about Alzheimer's Disease." The Lutheran Church (ELCA) has Lutheran Senior Life, which supports housing and health care facilities affiliated with the ELCA in Pennsylvania, one of which is for memory care. The United Methodists have a slew of congregational resources, including

Elizabeth Shulman's *Finding Sanctuary in the Midst of Alzheimer's.* Baptists, Congregationalists, Roman Catholics, Episcopalians, and others are joining in too. Sing from Memory, Abide, and Side by Side Respite are just a few of the programs that are spreading from church to church.

While congregations rally around the difficult issues created by dementia, they are discovering secular organizations that began working with those suffering from dementia, and their caregivers, decades ago. For instance, in 1994, Alzheimer's Disease International (ADI) launched World Alzheimer's Day on September 21 to celebrate the tenth anniversary of its founding. September 21 is also the day ADI releases its annual World Alzheimer Report. In 2012, it declared September as World Alzheimer Month.

Before ADI was established, the Alzheimer's Association was founded in 1980 in Chicago. It has become the largest nonprofit funder of Alzheimer's disease research in the world. It has over $310 million invested in more than 950 active best-of-field projects in forty-eight countries, and has launched three academic journals: *Alzheimer's & Dementia: The Journal of the Alzheimer's Association* in 2005; *Alzheimer's & Dementia: Diagnosis, Assessment & Disease Monitoring* in 2015; and *Alzheimer's & Dementia: Translational Research & Clinical Interventions,* also in 2015. More than six hundred communities in the United States now hold an annual Walk to End Alzheimer's to raise awareness and funds for Alzheimer's care, support and research, thanks to the Alzheimer's Association. Awareness of dementia in all of its facets is spreading from community to community.

Even the White House has gotten into the act. In July 2015, President Obama hosted the sixth White House Conference on Aging, a once-a-decade event sponsored by the Executive Office of the President of the United States, which makes policy recommendations regarding the aged. Out of this conference came the initiative known as Dementia Friendly America, which has grown into a national network of communities, organizations, and individuals seeking to ensure that communities across the US are equipped to support people living with dementia and their caregivers.

But for all the work that has been, and is being done, nationally and internationally, I am the most impressed with the quietly heroic efforts being made in the homes of those living with dementia. Sainthood comes in many forms. Spouses and children, and sometimes friends and neighbors, wear halos. The grace and strength and resolve of those who care for those who live with dementia is worthy of our commendation and support.

Remember my earlier comment about the stories I've been told about dementia? A couple of my friends took the trip of a lifetime—a seventy-four-day cruise from Fort Lauderdale, through the Panama Canal, around South America, and back to Florida again. In sharing their adventures with us (which were many) they mentioned some of the people they met along the way, who included a seventy-year-old Vietnamese woman named Huong Payson, who was traveling with her husband—as well as with her ex-husband.

This woman had been brought to America as a child after being adopted by a family from Philadelphia. She was raised and educated in the United States, married, and had three children. Somewhere along the line, she and her first husband divorced, and she later remarried. As things turned out, her first husband developed a form of dementia. They were still in touch with each other because of their children. Gradually, as he became increasingly disabled, she began to look out for him—with her second husband's support! When she and her second husband planned their cruise, they included her first husband so he would not be left alone.

On the last day of their trip, she wrote a poem about it—entitled "Here & There"—and gave it to my friends, who brought it home to me. The opening lines provide justification for the excursion:

> Too active for Nursing Home,
> Too old for Trek, for bike . . . alone!!!
> So, cruise around on a Holland America Grande Voyage,
> South America—Antarctica

Most of what follows is about the trip itself: crossing oceans, viewing glaciers, the rough seas, rain forests, wildlife, etc. But near the end she comes back to her opening sentiment with these words:

> Nursing Home must wait,
> Away on Holland America one should go . . .
> Some memorable trip for all . . .

As unconventional as their relationship might be, there is something wonderful about it. I hope that if I am ever diagnosed with dementia that I have a caregiver who will take me on a voyage. Or that my caretakers will at least postpone the nursing home or memory care until it is absolutely necessary.

Which brings me to the story I hope to tell with this book. In an earlier book I wrote, *Do Not Cast Me Away*, I sought to "demythologize" dementia. I tried to cover the major "bases" that people think about when confronted by dementia, in order to make it less daunting and to enable people to respond to it in helpful, meaningful, and faithful ways. I had congregations in mind, although much of what I wrote has proved helpful to individuals.

In this book, I intend to write for those caring for individuals who have dementia and how congregations and other groups can support them. Every facet of our society—church, synagogue, mosque, temple, neighborhood association, hospital, fraternal organization, and government at all levels—needs to gear up for this.

I am interested in interrelated questions: 1) How does one care for a person with dementia before institutional intervention occurs (nursing home, memory care, etc) and afterwards as well? And, 2) how does one care for that person's caregiver before any institutional intervention occurs, and afterwards as well? By the way, as you will read in what follows, an overwhelming number of people with dementia *will not have the option of institutional care*. They will live at home or in someone else's home. Hence the need for support for those helping them.

Pastoral care is part of my calling as a minister. In seminary we are taught to preach, teach, navigate our specific denomination's polity, and provide pastoral care as though we alone have the prerogative to do so. But the definition of pastoral care can be broadened to encompass any emotional, social, and spiritual support provided to another in Christ's name. All of us can be pastors in this sense. Especially when caring for those who cannot care for themselves. "Religion that God our Father accepts as pure and faultless is this: to look after orphans and widows in their distress and to keep oneself from being polluted by the world" (Jas 1:27). It can be argued that taking care of orphans and widows *is* the way to keep oneself from being polluted by the world.

Let me broaden pastoral care's definition even further: caring for others is not just something the ordained do—being pastoral is something everyone does when genuinely caring for another human being. This implies that not all caring is pastoral! Not all caring is genuine either.

Whether you are a pastor or not, or involved in a congregation or not, or are simply someone caring for a loved one with dementia, my prayer is that in the pages that follow you will find encouragement and support for your caring. May it be a memorable trip for you!

If you are part of a community of faith, my additional prayer is that you find it a dementia-friendly congregation.

Chapter One

Thoughts on Aging

Gray hair is a crown of splendor.

–Prov 16:31

He will renew your life and sustain you in your old age.

–Ruth 4:15

Aging is not for sissies. A member of a congregation I served in West Virginia gave an embroidered cushion to each of her friends when they turned seventy. It said, "Screw the Golden Years." A crude way to begin this conversation, perhaps, but doesn't it reflect our culture's attitude toward aging? Will Willimon says, "Just about everybody wants a long life; nobody wants to be old."[1] We live in a culture that glorifies youth, which was a wonderful thing when I was sixteen years old. Now that I am sixty-six years old, I'm not so sure!

The young are getting younger too. I know I do not understand "kids" these days. I mean, I *am* in my sixties. But I was talking with my son not too long ago—he is an early thirty-something public defender in a small town in East Tennessee—and he shared with me his frustration talking to a particular client, a nineteen-year-old man charged with several fairly serious crimes. During

1. Willimon, *Aging*, 2.

the course of the interview, my son said he was repeatedly unable to make out what point his client was trying to make. After finally stopping and asking, "What did you just say?," the response he got was that he (my son) was basically too old to "get it." Nothing like being irrelevant at thirty-three!

I think Martha Nussbaum is right when she argues that the aged are the subject of "widespread, indeed, virtually universal, social stigma."[2] Why is this? Why are older people commonly stereotyped as unattractive and useless? Agism really is prejudice and discrimination against the elderly, something that seems to be increasing in our digital age. The exasperated comments about all that is needed to fix grandmother's iPad is a twelve-year-old grandchild both extols the grandchild as a digital "native" and devalues the grandmother as a digital immigrant.

My guess is that the stigma toward the aged has to do with death. Not only are we an age-denying culture, we are a death-denying one as well. I mean, who enjoys thinking about their own mortality? Most of us are like the novelist William Saroyan, who wrote, "Everybody has got to die, but I have always believed an exception would be made in my case."[3]

In a cleverly entitled piece—"Thinking Botox with Barth"— Sara Mannen takes a step toward what she calls "a theology of beauty and aging" and declares: "My contention is that our culture's desire to erase the visible process of aging is another way we try to avoid our finite, limited bodies, and, ultimately, our deaths."[4] I agree with Mannen. In our culture, aging and death are inextricably linked together. We deny aging in order to keep death at bay. It functions as a sort of psychic buffer. Somewhere in the recesses of our minds, when we see an elderly person struggling to get around, we see ourselves in the same situation. We can't say to ourselves, "There but for the grace of God go I," because if we live long enough, there we will be![5]

2. Nussbaum and Levmore, *Aging Thoughtfully*, 10.
3. *New York Times*, "William Saroyan Is Dead," para. 2.
4. Mannen, "Thinking Botox with Barth," para. 8.
5. Swaim, "Why Ageism Happens."

This notion has been with us a long time. Even Shakespeare denigrated aging. In *As You Like It*, Jacques, an exiled nobleman, monologues about the seven ages of man: infant, schoolboy, lover, soldier, justice, pantaloon and old age. "All the world's a stage," he begins,

> and all the men and women merely players;
> They have exits and their entrances;
> and one man in his time plays many parts,
> His acts being seven ages.[6]

After commenting on each age, he concludes with this:

> Last scene of all,
> That ends this strange eventful history,
> Is second childishness and mere oblivion;
> Sans teeth, sans eyes, sans tastes, sans everything.[7]

Who wants to be "sans everything"?

It's true that "among the most difficult transitions you must make in life, the most traumatic changes occur after sixty-five: declining health, loss of independence, unemployment, loss of a spouse."[8] Yes, we may lose vigor, but that isn't the end of the story. Aging, growing old is just part of the story, yet there is so much more to tell!

While on sabbatical in Italy, I waited to cross a crowded street, and a man reached over and touched my white hair—actually pulled some of it through his fingers—and said, "Wisdom." The light changed and we went on. At first I thought it was creepy! Who touches another person's head? But I then decided he had given me a compliment: that with age comes a measure of wisdom and self-assurance. I know things now that I did not know earlier in life. I am not rattled by things that used to keep me up late at night, because I've been there and done that!

Life does not end at sixty-five or seventy. The joy of living—which includes simply knowing we are alive—can be with us no

---

6. Shakespeare, *As You Like It*, act 2, scene 7, lines 145–49.

7. Shakespeare, *As You Like It*, act 2, scene 7, lines 170–73.

8. Nussbaum and Levmore, *Aging Thoughtfully*, 41–42.

matter our age. There are no rules on this: the way we age, and the way we live as we age, are limitless. Years ago, one retired at sixty-four, pulled up a rocking chair on the front porch, and waited for the end. No more! Today, our churches and nonprofits and community organizations are full of older men and women putting their years of experience to work for others. So are our businesses.

My mother, at eighty-eight, is the "wheels" of her friendship circle, taking the "old folks" to their doctor appointments and making sure everyone "gets where they need to be." My father-in-law, also eighty-eight, is still an active participant on the board of a major manufacturing company. My favorite memories of hiking Mt. LeConte are those with a man in his eighties whose last trip up the mountain carrying a full backpack came at the age of eighty-nine. (He was disappointed when he was unable to make the trek at ninety, but he continued to man the "base" camp for our trips.) I know of a couple who moved from "up north" down to a lake in East Tennessee. After spending less than a month gazing at the spectacular view from their new front porch, they decided they were bored to tears, sold their retirement home, moved to Knoxville, and opened a restaurant.

The actor Michael Caine issued a statement that he had decided to retire at the age of ninety, and then later announced he was coming out of retirement for a role in a new Netflix series. Tony Bennett released a musical album of new material at the age of ninety-five. (He received seven Grammy nominations after being diagnosed with Alzheimer's in 2016, included winning one in 2019.) Betty White kept us laughing until her death at ninety-nine. Harlan Sanders started Kentucky Fried Chicken at sixty-two, and Warren Buffett is still running Berkshire Hathaway in his nineties.

In East Tennessee, retirees golf or fish or go boating whenever they can. Many of them hike and camp, travel abroad, and volunteer their services somewhere. A lot of seniors find part-time jobs, and it isn't always because they have to do so. Time and time again I have heard it said, "This time I get to work for myself." Or, "I always wanted to do this, now I can." Or, "It's time to give back to my community." Part-time jobs are just the start: a quarter of new entrepreneurs are aged fifty-five to sixty-four, and 54 percent of America's small business owners are over fifty. Seventeen percent are over sixty, and 4 percent are over seventy.

Older adults have an increasingly prominent presence on social media. Those aged fifty and over make up almost 20 percent of global social media users. Churchill Retirement Living (in the UK) has complied a list of the top ten "grandfluencers," beginning with Grandma Droniak, a ninety-three-year-old grandmother who got her social media start when she went online to share what she wants people to do at her funeral. She now has 8.8 million followers on TikTok. Ninety-five-year-old Helen Winkle has fun with her 3.2 million followers on Instagram. And at ninety-nine years of age, Iris Apfel has 2.6 million Instagram followers who love her fashion tips.[9]

Betty Friedan said, "Aging is not 'lost youth' but a new stage of opportunity and strength."[10] "Age is just a number," remarked Cicely Tyson. "Life and aging are the greatest gifts that we could possibly ever have."[11] The older people I know who live purposeful, meaningful lives agree with Edith Pearlman's commentary: "The ordinary experiences of aging alter and clarify your view of past, present, and future."[12] My mother-in-law says we all age, but we don't have to get old.

Even if we do get "old," no amount of aging, no infirmity, no illness, not even dementia, can alter the fact that whatever our age or whatever our health, we are created in the image of God. Genesis 1:27 reads: "So God created man in his *own* image, in the image of God created he him; male and female he created them." Admittedly, the exact meaning of the phrase is debatable, but there are no qualifiers in any of the primary biblical texts that utilize this notion. Nowhere does it say that we are created in the image of God because we are rational or moral, or have emotions or free will, or can speak a language, or are useful and productive, or are

9. Churchill Retirement Living, "New Top 10 'Grandfluencers.'"

10. Taylor, "Monday Motivation," para. 5.

11. Mitchell, "History," para. 2.

12. Ollivier, "Edith Pearlman," para. 8.

young, or anything else. There is a period at the end of Gen 1:27. We are created in the image of God. Period. As long as we are alive, no matter what condition we are in, in an undefined yet sacred way, we reflect the image of God. Even in old age.

Chapter Two

The Problem of Dementia

I thought, "Age should speak; advanced years should teach wisdom."

–JOB 32:7

WHEN I WAS A teenager, my father collapsed one morning while he was getting ready for work. I heard him fall. It wasn't difficult to figure out something was terribly wrong as he was moaning and spitting up blood. My mother telephoned for help while I held a garbage can for him to heave into. Anxiously, we waited for an ambulance to arrive. He was taken to a hospital and was diagnosed with a bleeding ulcer. After being transferred to a different hospital, he had surgery, which was followed by a long convalescence. When he returned home, we were prepared and ready for him, had a hospital bed set up, a side table for medications, "sitters" lined up to be with him at night, everything he might need. Gradually he got better and eventually returned to work.

His condition came on suddenly and very dramatically. There was no doubt he had a problem. There was no doubt medical intervention was necessary. There was no doubt that we (his family) were willing to do whatever it took to nurse him back to health, and we did. But what if his condition had not been so sudden and dramatic? What if we could not have put a finger on exactly what was happening to him? What if there had been no clear-cut interventions? Or if we had been uncertain as to how to care for him? Worst of all, what if we had lived with the dreadful notion that no matter what we did, or how lovingly we did it, he would never actually get better and that his illness could last for years?

I heard Bill Oglesby (professor of pastoral care at Union Theological Seminary in Richmond, Virginia, from 1952 until 1985) once say that the church is great at rallying around a person with an acute illness but lousy at helping a person with a chronic one. He might have said the same thing about families! In the early 1980s, when I was a seminarian, chronic conditions were things like heart disease, arthritis, or diabetes, illnesses that were persistent and long lasting. I do not remember a single conversation or lecture about dementia, either in graduate school or in seminary. In fact, a few years after seminary I talked with a professor at Columbia Theological Seminary, in Decatur, Georgia, who had designed a continuing education class in which he examined what he called the three *a*'s of pastoral care: aging, AIDS, and alcoholism. Neither of us thought to include a fourth *a* for Alzheimer's, and the subject was not brought up under "aging."

Chronic diseases by definition do not readily respond to treatment, even though there may be cycles of remission and relapse. The reality for those of us who want to be helpful to someone who is chronically ill is that we get tired and distracted. They aren't like the skinned knee that gets kissed and bandaged and forgotten about. Long-lasting illnesses are exhaustive. Other things get in the way. There are only so many casseroles that can be baked. How long can a person's name be kept on a prayer list? When people came to visit my father, he was visibly getting better; but how hard is it to see a person week after week without discernible improvement? How discouraging is it to hear the same thing from a caregiver over and over again: "Oh, she's about the same"?

Curious as to what I might have missed as a student, I thumbed through Howard Clinebell's *Basic Types of Pastoral Care*, which was our primary text in a seminary course on pastoral care. (The third edition was released in 2011, and I still consult it from time to time.) As I suspected, there is no listing of "memory" or "dementia" or "Alzheimer's disease" in the index. It is 496 pages long, and the topic of "aging" takes up just fifteen sentences. Two of those sentences are: "Demographic trends that point to increasing longevity carry huge challenges to caregivers." And, "More and more older people need care from family members as well as from all our social institutions, including churches."[1]

Talk about understatement! According to information on the Alzheimer's Association website, an estimated 6.7 million Americans age sixty-five and older are living with Alzheimer's. Seventy-three percent of them are age seventy-five or older. Almost two thirds of Americans with Alzheimer's are women. Black Americans are twice as likely to have Alzheimer's or other dementias than older White Americans, and older Hispanic Americans are 1.5 times more likely to the disease then their White counterparts. 1 in 3 seniors dies with Alzheimer's or another dementia. (It kills more than breast cancer and prostate cancer combined.) Deaths from Alzheimer's have more than doubled between 2000 and 2019. At age seventy, seniors living with Alzheimer's are twice as likely to die before age eighty than those who do not have the disease.

If these figures aren't startling enough, here are a few more, also from the Alzheimer's Association website: The lifetime risk for Alzheimer's at age forty-five is one in five for women and one in ten for men. Between 2020 and 2030, 1.2 million additional direct care workers will be needed for the growing population of people living with dementia. Over 11 million Americans currently provide unpaid care for people with Alzheimer's or other dementias, to the tune of 18 billion hours worth valued at $339.5 billion. You read that right: unpaid care. The average age for dementia caregivers is forty-nine. Incredibly, 25 percent of caregivers are between the ages of eighteen and forty-five, prime employment years. In 2015, Alzheimer's and other dementias cost our nation $226 billion. Estimates are that by 2050 the cost will soar to more than $1 trillion.

The US will have to quadruple the number of geriatricians to effectively provide for the number of people projected to have

---

1. Clinebell, *Basic Types*, 338–39.

Alzheimer's in 2050. Yet, according to an article published by the UNC School of Medicine on August 17, 2023, "the specialty is in decline."[2] The number of board-certified geriatricians has decreased for several decades even as the number of older adults has increased. The same article estimates that while there are currently about 7,500 licensed geriatricians in the US, we will need more than 30,000 geriatricians to meet the need.

The numbers are bleak: today, just 12 percent of nurse practitioners have special expertise in gerontological care. Less than 1 percent of registered nurses, physician assistants, and pharmacists identify themselves as specializing in geriatrics. Only 4 percent of social workers have formal certification in geriatric social work. Laura Reichen, director of Side by Side Respite Ministry in Greenville, South Carolina, says there is a "dementia tsunami" coming, and we are not ready for it.

None of the above comes close to covering the emotional and physical toll dementia takes. Who picks up the slack when the CEO of the largest employer in town develops dementia and jeopardizes everyone's job with reckless decisions he would never have considered just a few years earlier? What is the wife to do when her husband, in the early stages of dementia, cannot remember what his long-term care insurance policy is for and cancels it without telling her? What if the head of the local hospital or one of the chief surgeons begins to show signs of dementia?

Whatever else his book's shortcoming may be, Clinebell was absolutely correct that "more and more older people need care from family members as well as from all our social institutions, including churches."[3] Obviously, we need to get to work! But this is the kind of thing that needs thoughtfulness along with elbow grease. And perseverance. It will take a special kind of commitment from us, one that takes the long view. Helping a person with dementia, or helping a caregiver take care of a person with dementia, isn't a weekend mission trip. It isn't a series of church school classes an hour each week, or a conference from which we return

2. UNC School of Medicine, "Aging America."

3. Clinebell, *Basic Types*, 338.

as somewhat of an expert on whatever topic was presented. Caring for someone with dementia—enabling that person to feel he or she has not been cast aside or forsaken—enabling caregivers to feel they have not been cast aside or forsaken—takes sustained effort.

Volunteer work camps run on tools such as hammers and saws and levels, wielded by strong backs and arms and legs and good organizational structure. One or two experienced contractors can direct a host of willing laborers to accomplish a house-raising in just a few days. Not so with volunteering to help those with dementia. The tools needed are different and are sometimes not so obvious. Mostly it takes time. One person may help support a person with dementia and his or her caregiver for years. Michelle Cottle wrote an opinion piece for the *New York Times* in 2023, in which she stated, "Caregiving is essential work in an aging society, and at some point, most of us will have to confront its challenges." Her last sentence is "No one should have to face them alone."[4]

We need a plethora of intentionally dementia-friendly congregations, synagogues, mosques, temples, and community organizations, etc., to face the future of dementia care. We can do it. We must do it. *You* can do it. May you be inspired to take up the mantle of helping to care for those with dementia, and to support others (like yourself) that do as well.

4. Cottle, "You Shouldn't Have," para. 21.

Chapter Three

Just What Is Dementia?

The length of our days is seventy years or eighty,
if we have the strength;
Yet their span is but trouble and sorrow,
for they quickly pass, and we fly away.

—Ps 37:25

DEMENTIA HAS BEEN A recognized human condition for thousands of years. Plato and Hippocrates both theorized about the cause of mental decline.[1] Saint Isidore (AD 560–636), archbishop of Seville, used the term in his book *Etymologies*.[2] And dementia was recognized as a medical term in 1797 by a doctor in France.[3] Our grandparents might have called it "senility" or "hardening of the arteries."

YES, IT'S DEMENTIA, BUT WHAT EXACTLY DOES THAT MEAN?

It may be helpful to think of dementia as a disability, since it causes "long-term physical, mental, intellectual or sensory impairments"

1. Yang et al., "History of Alzheimer's Disease," para. 9.
2. Yang et al., "History of Alzheimer's Disease," para. 7.
3. Yang et al., "History of Alzheimer's Disease," para. 14.

17

that hinder "full and effective participation in society on an equal basis with others."[4] In other words, it is the result of disease (or injury), but it is also a social experience. What we are striving toward are ways to enable, rather than disable, those with dementia. We want a valid quality of life for as long as possible.

Along with making a home as safe as it reasonably can be for a person with dementia, it makes sense to know something about his or her condition in order to be as helpful as possible. While there are dozens of causes of dementia, there are only three "big" ones. (Or four or seven, depending on your source of information.) Below is a quick summary of the diseases you are most likely to encounter.

Alzheimer's disease (AD) is far and away the most common form of dementia, responsible for anywhere from 50 percent to 70 percent of all dementias. AD is caused by a buildup of proteins in the brain that affect how the brain cells transmit messages, a process first identified by Alois Alzheimer in 1906. The damage it causes is irreversible and progressive. It is thought to be responsible for as many as 500,000 deaths each year.

Early on, its symptoms are hardly noticeable. It comes on gradually. *On little cat feet.* Memory issues are noticed. Things like forgetting appointments, misplacing keys, struggling to find the right words, that sort of thing. Maybe one's balance isn't as good as it once was. Later on, though, there are disorientation and confusion. Perhaps even hallucinations, delusions, disturbed sleep, and obsessive—even aggressive—behaviors. Spatial awareness is sometimes compromised. Finally, serious physical and mental deterioration: difficulty eating and swallowing, incontinence, loss of speech, loss of mobility, increasing weakness, weight loss, and frailty.

Alzheimer's disease, though terminal, can last a long time. Estimates are that people live with it between three and eleven years after diagnosis. The middle stage is the longest, which is when it becomes apparent that more than forgetfulness is going

4. United Nations Department of Economic and Social Affairs, "Article 1—Purpose," para. 2.

on. The final stage lasts but one to two years. Obviously, the longer AD progresses, the more support a caregiver is going to need.

Vascular dementia (VaD) is the second most common type of dementia, caused by problems in the blood supply to the brain due to damaged or diseased blood vessels, a stroke, or "mini strokes" called transient ischemic attacks (TIAs). VaD isn't really a disease in and of itself, but is the consequence of the damage to the brain described above. Five percent to ten percent of all dementias are VaD, which typically lasts about five years.

The symptoms of vascular dementia depend on which area of the brain is affected, but generally include problems concentrating, slowed thought processes, trouble with short-term memory, and difficulty with everyday skills. There may be changes in personality and behavior, rapid mood swings, and compromised ability to make decisions and solve problems. There may also be speech or hearing issues.

There has been a lot of research into VaD, and several subtypes have been identified. Physicians refer to *subcortical vascular dementia* or *small vessel disease*. There is a condition called stroke-related dementia. And there is *multi-infarct dementia*. All three are caused by problems with blood vessels in our brains.

VaD is the one type of dementia impacted by lifestyle choices. Smoking and an unhealthy diet, combined with inactivity, may lead to an increased risk of stroke, hence, to vascular dementia. (Put away those cigarettes, and get up off the couch!) High blood pressure, diabetes, and atrial fibrillation all increase our chances for stroke.

Lewy body dementia (LBD), which accounts for 10 percent to 25 percent of all dementia, is caused by abnormal clumps of protein (called Lewy bodies, named for the neurologist who discovered them, Frederick Lewy) gathering inside brain cells, which they destroy. They tend to build up in those parts of the brain responsible for thought, movement, visual perception, and areas regulating sleep and alertness.

Symptoms may include visual hallucinations, disturbed sleep, fluctuations in alertness, slowed movement, difficulty walking, tremors, problems with balance, difficulties with swallowing, and bladder and bowel issues. Language and cognition are affected, and people may be at more risk to experience mood and behavior changes such as apathy, anxiety, depression, delusions, and paranoia. LBD can also affect blood pressure, heart rate, sweating, and digestion.

Lewy bodies are found in other brain disorders, too, including Parkinson's disease. LBD is sometimes misdiagnosed as Parkinson's because of the difficulty a person with LBD has with motor skills, or even as some sort of psychiatric illness, due to hallucinations and rapid changes in mood. Hallucinations often occur early in the disease process. People with LBD may regularly see animals or people or even shapes and colors that aren't there. It is thought that Lewy body dementia lasts anywhere from five to eight years after diagnosis.

These are the three major causes of dementia: Alzheimer's disease, vascular dementia, and Lewy body dementia. But there is one other major cause of dementia that deserves mention as a fourth major cause: *frontotemporal dementia (FTD)*, an umbrella term for a group of dementias that mainly affect the frontal and temporal lobes of the brain, which are responsible for personality, behavior, language and speech. Memory loss and concentration problems are common in the early stages. For some reason, it occurs more in people age forty to sixty than does Alzheimer's disease or Lewy body dementia.

There are two types of FTD—*behavioral variant FTD (bvFTD)* and *primary progressive aphasia (PPA)*. Symptoms of *behavioral variant FTD (bvFTD)* may include a lack of interest in things the person formerly enjoyed; inappropriate behavior; reduced empathy; difficulty focusing on tasks; obsessive or repetitive behavior; changes in behavior regarding food or drink; difficulty with planning, organizing, and decision-making; and a general lack of insight into themselves.

There are three types of primary progressive aphasia (PPA), all of which tend to affect language rather than behavior. Symptoms of the semantic variant or *semantic dementia (SD)* include difficulty remembering, finding, or understanding words; a grad-ual loss of vocabulary; and forgetting what common objects are and what they do. The non-fluent variant or *progressive non-fluent aphasia (PNFA)* is characterized by difficulty using speech, includ-ing forming sentences and using grammar correctly, and difficulty conducting conversations. Finally, the symptoms of the logopenic variant or *logopenic aphasia (LPA)* also include difficulty finding words, but unlike SD, people with early LPA are unlikely to forget the meaning of words or what common objects do.

In addition, there is also a condition known as *Huntington's disease*, a genetic disorder caused by a faulty gene, which leads to damage in the areas of the brain responsible for movement, learn-ing, cognition, and emotions. Folk singer Woody Guthrie and two of his children died of complications of Huntington's disease.

Creutzfeldt-Jakob disease is a rare brain disorder that leads to dementia. Many persons infected with the HIV virus suffer demen-tia later in life, known as AIDS dementia complex (ADC). About a third of people with *Parkinson's disease* will develop dementia, a type of dementia closely related to Lewy body dementia. There is alcohol-induced dementia, and dementia caused by *traumatic brain injuries*. All in all, there are more than two hundred types or causes of dementia, but more than likely if you meet someone with dementia, that person will be suffering from one of the three or four major causes discussed above.

My mother spent a career educating special needs children in southern Ohio. She once told me that given all that can go wrong with our fetal development, it's a wonder any of us function well. Given how many causes there are for dementia, it's a wonder any of us avoid it.

Caring for someone with dementia can be all consuming, emotionally, physically, and financially. Most of the families that deal with it do so without the means to afford nursing homes or even home health care. Long-term health insurance has proved to be a chimera. Governmental funds for elder care are virtually nonexistent. Families are on their own—unless they are able to become involved with a group of people seeking to help those with dementia. A church or a temple or a community group of some kind can make all the difference in the world.

Chapter Four

Making the Home "Safe"

Even to your old age and gray hairs I am he. I am he who will
sustain you. I have made you and will carry you; I will sustain you
and I will rescue you.

−Isa 46:4

After all the talk of the long-term commitment it takes to
help care for someone with dementia, there is something that one
or two people can do in a short period of time that can make a
significant difference, something that a congregation or community organization can do well. We can offer to help make a safer
home for both the one with dementia and the primary caregiver.
Most often, that primary caregiver will be a woman over the age
of sixty-five.

No two situations are alike, just as no two people are alike, yet
there are common themes that emerge when caring for a person
with dementia at home. Being in familiar surroundings is im-
mensely helpful to those with dementia. But being at home has it
own share of problems too. Here are a few of them, and almost all
of them can be modified.

Wherever possible, trip hazards need to be eliminated to
mitigate the possibility of a fall. People with dementia often have
problems with mobility and balance. They may "pace" and not notice hazards. A woman I often visited in West Virginia was proud

of her Oriental carpet collection. She had dozens of carpets. She even had smaller carpets placed on larger ones. She was constantly catching her cane on the edge of a Pakistani or Persian rug. To our great relief, she finally made it to a nursing home facility without breaking a hip. But she was one of the lucky ones!

Extension cords and low-level furniture are problematic. Some homes are built with electrical outlets in the middle of the floor. The intention is to provide current to a lamp placed by a couch or chair, but the outlet itself is exposed. Oftentimes the lamp cord is not tucked out of the way. If certain pieces of furniture are routinely bumped into before the onset of dementia, you can imagine what will happen after dementia sets in. Footstools and coffee tables can be deadly, as well as anything that rolls easily.

Steps and staircases are major headaches. Hardly anyone lives in a home completely void of stairs. "Modern" homes—those built in the 1960s—sometimes have spiral staircases. Or they are "split-level" with steps leading up and down. Older homes may have steps outside that lead down to a basement or furnace room. Not everyone can afford to install a lift, although this is one area where a crew from a church can make a significant difference for a person or family that needs one. Be cautious though: if a person with dementia lives alone, the controls to a lift may soon be beyond them.

Church groups are great at building wheelchair/walker ramps to entrances. We have a men's group that has done this. The width between handrails in the United States should be at least thirty-six inches (forty-eight inches is ideal). The minimum slope for hand-propelled wheelchairs should be one inch of rise for every twelve inches of length. In addition to ramps, some doorways can be widened, and railings can be added to hallways.

There's no end to the modifications that can be made to a home: grab bars for the bathrooms, elevated toilet seats, additional handrails for stairs that cannot be avoided, an adjusted hot water tank (with some sort of lock over the temperature control), better lighting, etc. The Alzheimer's Society has an online shop for daily living aids.

Many helpful things can be added to a home: large-faced LED clocks to tell time, labels on often-used items (either with words or pictures), locks on doorways that lead to dangerous places (like a basement or garage), and locks on cabinets that contain cleaning supplies. According to the AARP, more adults than children die from eating detergent![1]

If a person uses a walker, the single most dangerous moment he encounters is when he either goes into a home or out from a home by crossing a threshold, particularly if a step up or step down is involved. Think about it: he has to push the walker ahead of him, then momentarily let go of it in order to grasp the doorway to propel himself in or out, step across the threshold (up or down), then let go of the doorway to reach ahead to grasp the walker once again. He will be off balance, if only for a fraction of a second, but that may be enough for a fall. Additional handles, placed strategically on the door frame or close to the door fame, can make a world of difference. It is all about safety.

Since confusion and paranoia characterize some dementias, other kinds of questions need to be asked and addressed to ensure safety. Are there alarms in the home that can be monitored, such as those for a garage door opening or closing? Are there weapons in the house? Guns or knives? Don't assume that you know! After my father died, I was astonished at the number of guns we found in dressers and in closets. My mother had slept for who knows how long with a "goose" gun—a shotgun with a thirty-six-inch barrel—just a few feet from her head and never knew it was there!

Consider all possible weapons: antiques, collectibles, war souvenirs, hunting gear, etc. The Alzheimer's Association warns that locking or disabling a gun may not be enough, and that families should consider removing guns from the home to fully protect themselves and their loved one from an accident. Ammunition too.

The worry about guns in the house isn't primarily about homicide. It isn't about a person with dementia shooting someone else, although that happens. Rather, "the use of a firearm is the

---

1. Gobel, "Laundry Pods Killing," para. 2.

most common means of suicide among people with dementia; 73% of suicide deaths in those with dementia were due to a firearm in comparison with 50% of suicide deaths in people of all ages."[2]

There are dangerous power tools of all kinds—bench grinders, table saws, turning lathes, nail guns—this list is endless. Not to mention other potentially deadly items such as lawn mowers, chain saws, weed trimmers, gasoline, motor oil, paint thinner, etc. Hand tools are suspect too: screwdrivers, hammers, and chisels are but a few. Tool chests need to be locked. Storage buildings and garages must be secured. Church groups can help canvass homes and garages by looking for items that may be problematic.

An online Dementia Support Forum sponsored by the Alzheimer's Association in the UK included a helpful Q&A session on February 20, 2018, about dangerous tools. A registered user wrote in about a man with VaD (vascular dementia) who decided one day to "get rid of [a] small tree stump in the front garden." He asked for help unlocking the tool shed in order to get his chain saw. Luckily, there was no lubricant in the tank so it could not be used.

The explanatory comments by the registered user caught my attention. He wrote, "Sometimes I think that this early stage of dementia is doubly difficult as he is still able to do most things and I find it hard to stop him from doing stuff that can be dangerous or damaging." I hear the agony in his statement. How do we know what to do? Especially when the person we love is mostly his or her normal self.[3]

There are other things around the house to be considered. Better lighting helps reduce confusion. It also may decrease the possibility of a fall, especially on stairs or in the bathroom. Automatic light sensors, which come on when someone passes by, may be a good idea. (Any electricians in your church?) Are there working smoke detectors in the house? Do caregivers have extra keys to

2. Firth, "Preventing Gun Violence," para. 19.

3. Floria Tosca, "Using Dangerous Tools!," Alzheimer's Society Dementia Support Forum, Feb. 20, 2018, https://forum.alzheimers.org.uk/threads/using-dangerous-tools.107592/.

the house? Is one or two of them hidden outside in case they find themselves locked out?

We haven't gotten to the kitchen yet! Sharp-edged things reside in every drawer! More than 300,000 people visit an emergency room in the United States each year due to knife injuries. (Who knows how many of them suffer from dementia?) In addition to knives, there are box graters, shish kebab skewers, ice picks, and forks. Not to mention complicated gadgetry to operate, like can openers and toaster ovens, blenders and choppers.

What to do? The specifics will vary from kitchen to kitchen, of course, but the basic solution is this: declutter! Reduce the number of options of plates, pots, pans, cups, cutlery, etc. Go with nonbreakables wherever possible. A container that can seen through is always better than one that can't be seen through. You may need a gas-locking valve for the stovetop and a water overflow device for the sink. (And the bathtub.) There are even fridge alarms that alert you if a door has been left open, not to mention smoke and carbon monoxide alarms.

Let people help you make your house safer!

Then there is the garage. The car. When should someone step in and stop a person with dementia from driving? Honestly, losing the independence that driving a car gives is among the hardest complications of dementia that a person has to deal with. An "elder assessment" may help determine a person's ability to drive safely. What a congregation could do is organize rides to the various places a person with dementia may need to go. If this can be done on a regular basis, the sting of not driving may be lessened, to a worried caregiver's relief.

Chapter Five

Generally Speaking
Dementia and Communication

Those who are older should speak for wisdom comes with age.

–JOB 32:7

I think the most important thing I could share is just to meet them where they're at. . . . When you let go of who they've been or who you think they [should be], or who even you would like them to be, you can then really stay in the present and take in the joy and the love that is present and there for all that they are, not all that they're not.

–DEMI MOORE, ABOUT HER EX-SPOUSE BRUCE WILLIS, WHO WAS DIAGNOSED WITH FRONTOTEMPORAL DEMENTIA[1]

COMMUNICATION INVOLVES AN EXCHANGE of something—information or an emotion, an experience, a feeling or an idea. Something gets transmitted. That something may be verbal or nonverbal, written or visual, whatever. Regardless, an interaction occurs. When it happens between two people, there is reciprocity: something is sent, something is received. Good communication between people goes back and forth as a person acknowledges

1. Ibrahim, "Demi Moore Speaks Out," paras. 5–6.

what she hears, or feels, from another person and replies in kind. Except, of course, when it doesn't. Except when one of the participants has dementia.

Knowing a bit about the kind of dementia a person has can greatly facilitate communicating with that person, which is why a summary of the types of dementia was presented in the previous chapter. There are plenty of practical things each of us can do to communicate with and support a person with dementia.

I've found it helpful to remember that dementia is a progressive disorder. It unfolds over time, which means there is time for family and friends and congregations to gear up to be helpful. It isn't an acute illness but a chronic one. A person isn't told he has Alzheimer's disease in the morning and forgets who he is that afternoon. Most of the experts on dementia consider it to have three stages, although some groups talk about seven stages. The three-stage camp refers to early, middle, and late.

In the *early stage* of dementia, a person will start to experience problems that affect his or her everyday living. He or she may notice these early changes themselves, or they may first be recognized by their family, friends, or colleagues. In the *middle stage*, the mild problems that the person first experienced become more pronounced and start to affect his or her ability to live without some form of support. In the *late stage* of dementia, the changes in the person become more pronounced to the point where he or she is unable to live independently. But before a person can no longer live independently, a lot of living and a lot of caring can take place.

If a person has *Alzheimer's disease*, remaining socially connected by including him or her in familiar activities can be very helpful. And why not? Early- and middle-stage AD may last years. Having dementia does not make someone a pariah. By all means, take them to church and Bible study, to the weekly card game, or to watch the Tennessee Volunteers on television with friends. What this takes mostly is time. You may not get quite the same return on your efforts as in the past, but with early into middle Alzheimer's, they know, they're aware, they appreciate your effort and your presence. The caregiver will certainly appreciate the break.

If a person has *vascular dementia*, remember to speak in short, simple sentences. Break complex tasks down into smaller steps, which are easier to follow, one at a time. (If you have a child or grandchild with ADD, you have had plenty of practice with this!) Try to avoid something like, "Go upstairs and change your clothes—put on something nice—we're leaving for church in about thirty minutes." Choices can be significant stressors for people with dementia, as are time constraints. And no one likes being told what to do!

Lewy body dementia is often accompanied by wild mood swings. Knowing this, keep your voice low and melodic, and your movements calm and controlled. Keep it slow. LBD is known to also affect language and cognition. "In conversations, persons with LBD experience difficulties in turn-taking, topic initiation, entering conversations and keeping up with the conversational tempo."[2] Keep it slow when talking with someone who has Lewy body dementia. In fact, keep it slow no matter what type of dementia a person has. Not childish, just slow.

In *frontotemporal dementia*, unlike other types of dementia, memory loss and concentration problems are less common in the early stages. Communication can be less guarded, because his memory in intact, but his ability to respond is impaired. Don't get frustrated waiting for him to speak. For a while, with a person I knew with *primary progressive aphasia*, we used an iPad to talk back and forth. Sometimes we just used paper and pen. But as his illness advanced, he simply withdrew from all attempts to communicate, sitting quietly for hours by himself in a chair.

The DementiaUK website has this to say about communicating with a person with dementia, understanding that communication itself is fundamental to our ability to express ourselves, and our relationships with other people:

> We communicate not only through our words but also our body language, facial expressions and tone of

2. Lindeberg et al., "Conversations in Dementia," abstract, under "What Is Already Known on the Subject."

voice—but people with dementia may have challenges with all of these forms of communication.

They may experience:

- Difficulty finding the right words, and sometimes using the wrong word
- Difficulty pronouncing words
- Muddling words, such as "aminal" rather than "animal"
- Problems following a conversation, especially in a noisy environment
- Difficulty understanding humour or sarcasm
- Difficulty reading other people's emotions or understanding their behaviours
- A tendency to repeat themselves
- Fluctuating concentration and communication abilities, often caused by tiredness or ill health
- Stress caused by struggling to make their views, needs and feelings known[3]

The same website provides tips for communicating with a person with dementia. Keep in mind that a person with dementia can often understand far more than they can communicate, so always try to involve them in your conversation. Small changes in your approach can make a big difference. It is helpful to:

- Stop what you're doing and focus entirely on the person
- Limit distractions
- Say their name when talking to them
- Touch their arm, if they feel comfortable with this
- Smile
- Speak slowly, clearly and in short sentences
- Use simple and straightforward language
- Listen carefully with empathy and understanding
- Give the person plenty of time to answer
- Maintain appropriate eye contact
- Be specific, try not to use pronouns such as "he" or "she" when talking about others; use their name instead

3. Dementia UK, "Tips for Communicating," under "How Dementia Affects Communication."

- Use gestures to act out what you're saying—for example, by miming drinking a cup of tea or putting on your shoes
- Use pictures to explain what you're saying, such as an image of a car or a photo of where you're going
- Avoid open-ended questions or offering too many choices
- Use visual timetables—where you use photos or images to show what will happen at various times of the day[4]

I realize the above, as helpful as it is, is a lot to remember. Here is a shorter list of "don'ts" compiled from advice by Alzheimer's San Diego:

Don't reason
Don't argue
Don't confront
Don't remind them they forgot
Don't question recent memory
Don't take it personally

The flip-side of "don'ts" is things to do, like:

Give short, one-sentence explanations
Allow plenty of time for comprehension
Avoid insistence
Agree and/or distract
Respond to feelings rather than the words
Be patient
Practice 100% forgiveness[5]

When I visit a person with dementia, even now, I almost always have to remind myself of these tips. So much of our communication is flippant. We use slang and all sorts of verbal shorthand. We don't make consistent eye contact. Being "in the moment" with anyone takes effort, much less with a dementia patient.

The biggest hindrance I experience to being in the moment with a person with dementia is the other people nearby. A caregiver

4. Dementia UK, "Tips for Communicating," under "Tips for Communicating."

5. Alzheimer's San Diego, "Do's and Don'ts."

is always easier to speak with than the person with dementia. He or she may even answer for the patient. If I am not careful, I find myself looking back and forth, from person to person, which interferes with my ability to communicate clearly with the one I am there to see.

Virtually everyone's preference is to age at home. The only person I have known who preemptively chose someplace else was a woman from Ashland, Kentucky. Once she was diagnosed with Alzheimer's disease, she sold off her home and her car and moved into an assisted living facility that had a nursing home "wing" attached to it. It all happened so quickly, none of us knew what was going on. When I spoke with her about it, she told me matter-of-factly that she didn't want anyone to have to make decisions for her, so she made them while she still could. After getting over the shock of it all, her children were relieved and grateful.

What she did was save them from becoming primary caregivers. The next chapter looks at just what that might entail.

Chapter Six

Who Is a Caregiver?

Each of you should look not only to your own interests, but also to the interests of others.

—PHIL 2:4

ANTHEA ROWAN, IN AN article that appeared in a 2023 issue of *Psychology Today*, wrote, "Dementia starts in the head and then hijacks the body."[1] What she also could have said is that dementia hijacks the caregiver too! For most of the people in the congregations I have served who became dementia caregivers, the disease came on so slowly that they were unaware they were becoming caregivers until they actually were. They were quietly hijacked.

How do you know this has happened to you? When you suddenly realize you cannot go somewhere you'd like to go because you cannot figure out how to have your loved one taken care of in your absence. Or because you are unwilling to let someone "sit" with your loved one because you've realized the things you do to keep life at an even keel are too complicated to be briefly shared.

There may be in this instance—becoming hijacked—what C. S. Lewis would call "a severe mercy"[2] in that the caregiver has more or less had time to ease into this role, but what a task! It can be so stressful such caregivers have been called "the invisible

1. Rowan, "Dreadful Physical Symptoms," para. 22.
2. Vanauken, *Severe Mercy*.

second patient."[3] Pastors and congregations (not to mention physicians) simply must pay attention to caregivers.

Who are our caregivers? Two thirds of Alzheimer's disease patients are cared for at home by family members, neighbors, or friends. Since they aren't paid, economists who study this sort of thing refer to them as *informal* caregivers. (This isn't meant to be condescending, although it sounds like it is!) An astonishing 41 percent of caregivers are between the ages of fifty and sixty-four (peak earning years). Sixteen percent are under thirty-five.

It is estimated that as many as 1.4 million children under the age of eighteen provide care for an adult relative, a parent or grandparent.[4] I can think of at least one situation in every congregation I have served where an adult child has more or less sacrificed his or her career/relationships/everything to live at home to take care of Mom or Dad, or both.

The vast majority (66 percent) of dementia caregivers are women, 19 percent of whom had to quit work to become a caregiver or quit because their caregiving became too burdensome. Adult children, more so than spouses, are likely to be caregivers. However, to be fair, while more daughters provide care for older adults with dementia, spouses provide more hours of care per month than daughters.[5] A worrisome statistic is that about one in three caregivers is sixty-five years of age or older: approaching the time when they might need care themselves. And let's not forget those who are "sandwiched" between caring for children under eighteen as well as caring for aging parents. Then there are those who watch after aging parents while raising grandchildren. Life really isn't fair sometimes!

Formal caregivers, who receive pay for the care they provide, and who have some kind of certification and training, come in as many shapes and sizes as informal caregivers do. Formal caregivers provide "outpatient" or "home-based" care. They include social

3. Brodaty and Donkin, "Family Caregivers," abstract.

4. For the most recent statistics, see https://www.caregiveraction.org/resources/caregiver-statistics.

5. ASPE, "Profile of Older Adults," para. 9.

workers, home health aides, registered nurses, nurses' aides, medical doctors, occupational therapists, physical therapists, speech therapists, and hospice nurse practitioners. I'm sure I've left someone out.

Formal care is both home based and community based. Home based means the care is provided at home. The care comes to you, so to speak. Community based refers to care provided by trained staff at places like adult day care centers. The division between the two isn't as neat as this distinction might seem. Though formal caregivers come into the home, the bulk of the care is still informal. The same is also true for community-based care. Even if the person with dementia eventually goes into a "home," the informal care for that person does not cease.

When the disease is in its early stage, people function independently. As previously stated, it is hardly noticed at all. The caregiver's role is mainly to provide love and support, and to help plan for the future. The caregiver and the person with dementia have the opportunity to make decisions together, to research and take advantage of available treatments, and to learn about and begin to access local support services. Mostly, life goes on as usual.

Later on, in the middle stage, caregivers have to take on greater responsibility. The one being cared for may experience depression, anxiety, irritability, repetitive behaviors, etc. As the disease progresses, other changes may occur, including sleep changes, physical and verbal outbursts, and possibly wandering. Eating, dressing, and grooming will become more challenging. Decisions about driving have to be made. Financial matters come to the fore. Dangerous items around the house, especially guns, need to be addressed.

The late stage of Alzheimer's disease is every person's nightmare. Difficulty eating and swallowing; needing assistance walking; needing full-time help with personal care; being vulnerable to infections, especially pneumonia, is just a start. I like what the Alzheimer's Association has to say about the role of a caregiver during this stage:

Your role as a caregiver focuses on preserving quality of life and dignity. Although a person in the late stage of Alzheimer's typically loses the ability to talk and express needs, research tells us that some core of the person's self may remain. This means you may be able to continue to connect throughout the late stage of the disease.

At this point in the disease, the world is primarily experienced through the senses. You can express your caring through touch, sound, sight, taste and smell. For example, try:

Playing his or her favorite music
Reading portions of books that have meaning for the person
Looking at old photos together
Rubbing lotion with a favorite scent into the skin
Brushing the person's hair
Sitting outside together on a nice day.[6]

This sounds so serene and bucolic we are tempted to forget there are very difficult challenges to being a dementia caregiver. "Of Alzheimer's caregivers, 58% of participants reported extremely high stress levels. Over time, high levels of frustration and stress may lead to caregiver burnout. This can cause feelings of physical, mental, and emotional exhaustion."[7]

Care becomes increasingly complex and more and more time consuming as Alzheimer's disease or other dementias progress. It can be *all* consuming: everything else and everyone else takes a backseat! The number one cause of dementia caregiver burnout is isolation, something we will talk about in the next chapter.

Still, there are rewards. In an article written for the *New York Times* in 2011, Paula Span notes, "Along with what's called 'caregiver burden,' gerontologists and psychologists use the phrase 'caregiver gain' to reflect the fact that this role, which often exacts such high costs, can bring rewards." In addition to caregiving gains self-described as "feelings of personal satisfaction" or "increased

6. Alzheimer's Association, "Late-Stage Caregiving," under "Your Role as Caregiver."

7. Grey, "Alzheimer's, Caregiving, Managing Frustration," paras. 6–7.

family closeness"—that sort of thing—it was surprisingly discovered that dementia caregivers "can walk faster [and] recall more words on a memory test."[8]

It seems that for some caregivers there are quantifiable benefits: "Caregivers, however stressed, may be stronger and stay stronger than women of the same ages who don't undertake those tasks" associated with caregiving.[9] Caregiving requires you to move around a lot, to be up on your feet, moving, bending, lifting. Caregivers monitor medications, juggle schedules, take on financial responsibilities, interact with health care providers, and keep up with household chores and other family responsibilities. It is true that "caregivers are not invariably beaten down by their responsibilities."[10]

The ninety-something wife of a man with dementia, whom I see often, tells me over and over how lucky she is to be able to care for her husband at this point in their life together. I think she means it! Of course, it's a burden. But, as she says, "There's always something!" If it wasn't this, it would be something else.

Caregivers—hijacked or not—are the most important link in a dementia patient's chain of support. Medical science is beginning to quantify just how valuable they are. An article that appeared on the NeurologyLive website in 2023 details "multi-time series longitudinal study" findings that "caregivers' perceived reciprocity may reduce the number of behavioral symptoms a patient with Alzheimer's disease and related dementias (ADRD) experiences."[11] In other words, caregivers really do impact both the environment and the behavioral symptoms in patients with Alzheimer's. Compassionate caregivers are worth their weight in gold.

This study indicates that it isn't just the nuts and bolts of caregiving that helps, but that engaging "in a pleasant noncare activity with the patient" makes a difference.[12] Church and community vol-

8. Span, "Caregiving's Hidden Benefits," para. 8.
9. Span, "Caregiving's Hidden Benefits," para. 9.
10. Span, "Caregiving's Hidden Benefits," para. 9.
11. Ciccone, "Caregivers [sic] Perceived Reciprocity," para. 1.
12. Ciccone, "Caregivers [sic] Perceived Reciprocity," para. 5.

unteers who provide informal non-care activity can be as valuable as many formal caregivers. There is plenty of time for it: "Well over half (57%) of family caregivers of people with Alzheimer's and related dementias provide care for four years or more."[13]

13. CDC, "Caregiving," para. 5.

Chapter Seven

The Isolation of Caregiving

Be kind and compassionate to one another, forgiving each other,
just as in Christ God forgave you.

—EPH 4:23

THERE ARE ENORMOUS PROBLEMS faced by dementia caregivers on a daily basis. As I have written before, sainthood comes in all shapes and sizes with all sorts of tribulations. Below are some of the problems at-home caregivers face. Each one contributes to the sense of isolation a caregiver can come to feel.

LONELINESS

Quite naturally, the family member with dementia becomes the family's center of attention. Gradually, the world begins to revolve around that one person. Family, neighbors, and friends offer to help—with that person. People bring food especially made—for that person. Pastors come to visit—that person. Neighbors stop by to see—that person. You get the picture: the primary caregiver of—that person—can become wallpaper in the background. Or, at least, he or she can feel that way. Loneliness may be the hardest, most difficult issue facing a dementia caregiver.

Loneliness is that feeling of isolation or lack of connection with people and places that are important. (Not to mention the frayed and fraying relationship with the one being cared for!) A caregiver is not as free to get out and see people as before. The monotony of the daily struggle can be stultifying. The walls can close in. There can be very little to look forward to, except more of the same. I know a woman who said the highlight of her day was getting the mail: virtually the only time she went outside the home. Unlike a terminal illness such as cancer, which can last months, dementia can last years.

Psychologists write about different kinds of loneliness (as if one kind isn't enough): emotional loneliness, which is the absence of meaningful relationships; social loneliness, which is the absence of social connections; and existential loneliness, which is the feeling of loneliness that comes from separation from all that has meaning and purpose in the broader world. A savvy congregation can make a world of difference to a person struggling with any sort of loneliness.

FINANCIAL WORRIES

Financial worry is a great cause of loneliness, due to the way our society handles its money matters, which is sort of like an addiction: something we don't talk about. Nothing is more isolating than not knowing what to do or where to turn. The cost of dementia care is depressingly high. I heard a news feature on NPR that said, "First, Alzheimer's takes away a person's memory. Then it takes their family's money."[1]

There are plenty of things to find out: Whose name is on the checking account and on the savings account? How many accounts are there? Is there a mortgage? Is there a car? Are there insurance policies? Who are beneficiaries? Are there credit cards? Where are all the important documents? Is there a safe? Does anyone know the combination to it? What about a safe-deposit box? My father, unbeknownst to me, kept amazingly large amounts of cash in

1. Hamilton, "Big Financial Costs," para. 1.

old suitcases. Don't overlook the possibility of money stashed in mattresses!

Furthermore, is there a will? Or a living will? A do-not-resuscitate order? Is there a family attorney? The most important document (other than a will) to have is a power of attorney, because it provides authorization to act on behalf of the person with dementia. It should be durable (meaning it takes effect immediately and indefinitely) and general (as opposed to limited), allowing control over a broad range of legal, financial, and medical matters. Be aware that durable power of attorney can be revoked, in some states easily so. It's a good idea for a caregiver taking on financial responsibilities through durable power of attorney to review its ins and outs with an attorney.

MEDICATIONS

Every dementia sufferer's home eventually looks like a small pharmacy. There are canes, walking frames, rollators, wheelchairs, scooters, raised toilet seats, shower stools, grab rails, boxes of adult pull-up pants, urinals, bedpans, hand sanitizers, and cleaning wipes. There is usually a hospital bed with some sort of mobile tray table. And there are lots and lots of medications. Too many, in fact. Way too many. Managing the medications for individuals with dementia can be confusing and difficult, especially if the person being cared for is resistant, belligerent, or both.

Keeping up with medication is an ornery task. Caregivers need to ask questions about them. For instance, is it really necessary for a man with middle- to late-stage Alzheimer's disease, who is having trouble swallowing, to continue to take that statin drug he was prescribed umpteen years ago? And what about those heart meds? An involved physician—hopefully a geriatrician—can be asked to review the list of medications being taken by a person with dementia and provide guidance.

Regardless, a list of medications ought to be kept, along with a schedule of when each is to be taken, even noting side effects (if any can be discerned). SingleCare has a template that can be downloaded and used.[2] It suggests putting supplements first, then over-the-counter medications, then prescription drugs. Almost always, all medications will eventually need to be stored in a locked cabinet somewhere. Stories of medicine "going missing" are legion, and while there are many reasons for this, we do not need to be naive about the lure of certain drugs on display in a sick person's room.

BATHING AND DRESSING

Helping someone with dementia take a shower may be the single most physically and emotionally difficult thing a caregiver can do. Sometimes the person is afraid of the water. Or of the steam from the water. Or of the sound it makes. It is possible that instead of feeling good or refreshing, they fear it will be painful. It may actually be painful! Or they may just be embarrassed.

A suggested routine to establish before the bath is to get everything ready: soap, washcloth, towels, baby shampoo (it doesn't sting the eyes), etc. Is the anti-slip rubber mat in the right place? Are the safety bars sturdy? Is there need for a shower chair? Or a handheld showerhead? Make sure the room is warm and the water temperature is comfortable. Never leave a person alone in a tub or shower. If the temperature is accidentally turned too hot, they may not be able to turn it off. Bath time may very well be a two-person job. Two or three times a week may have to suffice. (Washing a person's hair in a sink may be easier than in a tub.) There is nothing wrong with simple sponge baths.

Dressing afterwards can also be a chore, but doing things like laying out clothes—in the order they should be put on—can help a person dress himself on his own. Laying out the clothes limits the number of layers of clothing a person may put on, as knowing when to stop getting dressed can be as difficult as knowing how to get dressed in the first place. Loose-fitting items, with elastic

2. See https://www.singlecare.com/blog/medication-list-template/.

waistbands, are always winners, along with Velcro and slip-ons instead of laces.

GROOMING

Everyone feels better when they are clean and put together. After the bath comes grooming. Helping people with Alzheimer's disease brush their teeth, shave, put on makeup, and get dressed can help them feel more like themselves. A caregiver may have to show a person how to brush his or her teeth. Go slowly, step by step. It may be helpful to brush your teeth and comb your hair at the same time. If the person has dentures, they will need to be cleaned too. A dentist specializing in treating dementia patients would be a plus. Some cities have mobile dentists who will come to you.

Encourage a woman to wear makeup if she has always used it. If needed, help her put on powder and lipstick, but avoid eye makeup. Encourage a man to shave, and help him as needed. Use an electric razor for safety. Or take the person to the barber or beauty shop on a regular basis. If a person has always used certain brands of perfume or cologne or aftershave, etc., stick with it. The familiarity may be comforting. Grooming can be hard enough without having it sabotaged over something that can be avoided.

Keeping the person's nails clean and trimmed can be an adventure, especially the feet. Like taking a shower, trimming nails may be frightening or painful. Soaking the fingers and toes in warm, soapy water to soften them sometimes helps. Talking to them, watching a show, something to provide a distraction may work. In the end it may be necessary to see a podiatrist.

Once the above has been handled (or not!), how much time and energy are left over for the caregiver's own needs?

Chapter Eight

Sundowning and Wandering

Whatever you did for the one of the least of these brothers of
mine, you did it for me.

–MATT 25:40

THE SIMPLEST CHORES OF daily living with a person with dementia
can be wearing enough, but there are two issues that rise above
the others in both degree and severity: sundowning and wandering. Informal caregivers may very much feel "in over their heads"
and in need of professional help dealing with them. All the more
reason for plenty of support from their community of friends and
faith!

SUNDOWNING

Sundowning is a very real, authenticated, and documented condition experienced by some people with dementia. It is estimated to
afflict as many as 20 percent of people with Alzheimer's disease.
Caregivers of a person with sundowners, or sundown syndrome,
dread the approach of evening. While the rest of us are winding
down from a day's activities, the restlessness, agitation, or confusion experienced by someone with Alzheimer's disease gets worse.
There may even be hallucinations.

No one knows why this happens. The best guest is that Alzheimer's disease affects a person's biological clock, confusing their sleep-wake cycle. Trey Todd, a neuroscientist at the University of Wyoming, says: "Nurses will talk about it like almost a light switch."[1] It begins about the same time in the late afternoon/early evening and lasts anywhere from three to five hours. It can be terribly disruptive! In fact, the same article that cites Trey Todd's comment goes on to say that sundowning "is often what drives families to seek full-time professional care for their loved ones."[2]

The Alzheimer's Caregivers Network lists the following behaviors commonly associated with sundowning:

- Pacing
- Rocking in a chair
- Wandering
- Violence
- Shadowing
- Crying
- Insomnia
- Yelling

These behaviors listed above seem to go hand in hand with the following emotions:

- Sadness
- Anxiety
- Fear
- Agitation
- Restlessness
- Irritability

The end result is often (not always) unfortunate mental states, such as:

- Confusion
- Paranoia
- Hallucinations and delusions[3]

1. McKeever, "Why Evenings," para. 2.
2. McKeever, "Why Evenings," para. 4.
3. Alzheimer's Caregivers Network, "Caregiver's Guide," under

Sundown syndrome looks different for everyone who experiences it; symptoms can stop abruptly, change, or fade over time. It can be very difficult for both informal and formal caregivers to manage.

In a few cases, symptoms persist throughout the night, making it hard for people with Alzheimer's disease to fall and stay asleep. A disrupted sleep routine often means they and their caregivers will not be getting enough rest to function well during the daytime. It is hard enough being a caregiver without also being sleep deprived.

Studies have shown that sundowning behavior in people with Alzheimer's disease can increase when they sense frustration, anxiety, or stress from their caregivers. Be patient, but most importantly, recognize when you need a break and rest. Your sleep is just as important as your loved one's is. You can't help them cope with sundowning symptoms if you're both exhausted. If ever there was a time to call on someone for help, after a stretch of dealing with sundowning, that is the time!

Amazingly enough, sundowning has been a named condition since the 1940s, when it was referred to as "nocturnal delirium."[4] Unfortunately, treating it is still largely guesswork. Still, there are a variety of techniques that can be tried. For instance, bright-light therapy—like the kind used for seasonal affective disorder or jet lag—seems to help some of those suffering from Alzheimer's. Do this by opening window coverings during the day for maximum exposure to bright light. At dusk, close the window coverings and turn lights on (LED brights) to eliminate residual shadows caused by the late daylight.

Caregivers should consider:

- Incorporating calming activities into the evening, like doing a puzzle, having a snack, or enjoying a phone call with a loved one.
- Minimizing loud background noises, and especially turn down loud television programs. If needed, create

---

"Recognizing Sundown Syndrome and Its Symptoms."

4. Khachiyants et al., "Sundown Syndrome," "Introduction," para. 3.

low, calming background noise (like white noise) to help to lessen the impact of loud and sudden noises.

- Minimizing clutter in rooms and/or the number of people in the room. (Early evening is *not* a good time for the church fellowship committee to visit.)
- Monitoring screen time on all devices as certain content can be upsetting for people with dementia.

It is also suggested that incorporating these daily behaviors into your loved one's life may (somewhat) lessen the affect of sundowning:

- Maintain a predictable routine for bedtime, waking up, meals, and activities, which helps your loved one know what to expect throughout the day, which comforts them.
- Get daily outside physical activity and exercise.
- Eliminate caffeine and alcohol, especially in the late day.
- Keep daytime naps short and earlier rather than later in the day.[5]

WANDERING

About 60 percent (three out of five) of people with dementia, including those with Alzheimer's disease, will experience wandering. Not just walking: wandering. Walking or pacing—a lot—may be a way to relieve anxiety. This may occur when a senior with dementia is trying to find someone or something. It may also be the result of discomfort, anxiety, or even fear.[6]

"If a person is confused because of memory changes, and the environment becomes uncomfortable, they may attempt to leave the situation to get away from the discomfort," says Andrea Denny, outreach, recruitment and engagement core leader for the Knight Alzheimer Disease Research Center in St. Louis, Missouri. "This desire to escape the overwhelming stimuli may cause what we call

---

5. See Alzheimer's Association, "Sundowning," for the most current ideas.
6. Samuels, "Dementia and Wandering," para. 1.

wandering."[7] While people with dementia often leave with a goal or destination in mind, they may forget directions, encounter an obstacle in their planned route, or realize the place they're trying to reach is imaginary or inaccessible. Unfortunately, wandering, like sundowning, is something we just don't know enough about. Except that it happens.

Wandering is a serious concern for families, caregivers, and law enforcement officials and is sometimes called "elopement" or "critical wandering." It can lead to what is known as a "missing person incident" or a "silver alert."

This occurs when the whereabouts of a person with dementia is unknown to the caregiver, and the person with dementia is not in the expected location. Because dementia impairs a person's ability to recognize that they are in danger or to independently take action to return home safely, missing incidents can pose a serious threat to the personal safety of a person with dementia or Alzheimer's disease. Research indicates that about half of those who are not found within twenty-four hours risk serious injury or death.

Wandering—like sundowning—is underreported because so many people with dementia live alone. Estimates range from one in seven to one in four people with dementia live alone in the United States. Congregations can keep track of members with health problems (like dementia) through a simple phone tree. If someone doesn't answer, go check up on them. Or call 911 to request a wellness check. The important thing is being in touch with them.

Wandering most commonly occurs in the middle or later stages of dementia, but don't rule it out in the early stage. Nearly 50 percent of seniors who wander will suffer a fall, fracture, injury, or some type of elemental exposure, according to a 2016 assessment of wandering behaviors in the International Journal of Geriatric Psychiatry. This is evidently due to the confusion, disorientation, and decreased physical coordination brought on by the disease.[8]

---

7. Samuels, "Dementia and Wandering," para. 2.
8. Ali et al., "Risk Assessment," abstract, under "Results."

A Place for Mom lists "12 Ways to Prevent Dementia Wandering," beginning with "Provide supervision."[9] Easier said than done! Early on, of course, a person can be alone for short periods of time without worry. But later on, a neighbor or a church friend—someone—will need to be present in order for the primary caregiver to have time to run errands or go to work or just rest up.

It is also thought that "neutral door coverings and floor mats in front of doorways reduce exit-seeking behaviors." A Place for Mom even recommends placing removable curtains or paint or wallpaper in such a way as to obscure entries and exits.[10]

Other suggestions include keeping "trigger" items out of sight, such as car keys or a hat and gloves. Of course, alarms, locks and motion sensors can let you know when a person with dementia is on the move. One family I know has an electric eye device that beeps a warning if someone walks too close to the front door. You can try things like warning bells on doors, childproof covers on doorknobs, and sliding bolts installed either above or below eye level.

Nighttime wandering often goes hand in hand with sundowning. Be prepared: it will happen. I can't tell you how often I've heard a caregiver call a loved one "Houdini." It can be vital to have a recent, close-up photo on hand, along with up-to-date medical information to give to police should that be necessary, as well as a list of people to call for help.

We can all rest a little easier knowing that most wandering does not involve an "escape." Sometimes a loved one is simply up and about at all hours of the night. It is hard to know what to call this, wandering or sundowning or a combination of both. One of our members told me of waking up at 4:30 a.m. and finding her husband fully dressed sitting in a chair beside the bed. He wasn't trying to go anywhere, but he wasn't in bed where he was supposed to be. She said she didn't know how he did it, as he is normally

9. In Samuels, "Dementia and Wandering."

10. Samuels, "Dementia and Wandering," "12 Ways to Prevent Dementia Wandering," item 2.

unable to get himself completely dressed. She added, "Who knows what's going on in his head?!"

Chapter Nine

Every Rope Becomes Frayed

He gives strength to the weary
and increases the power of the weak.

—Isa 40:29

If there is anything that gives nightmares to what may already be the dark night of 24/7 caregiving, it is the thought of illness to the caregiver herself. What happen if she gets sick? What will happen to the one being cared for? This is a huge issue! If illness weren't bad enough, there is caregiver burnout to worry about too.

The Caregiver Space is an online community of caregivers that provides "a place to ask questions, share experiences, get real answers, or just get things off your chest."[1] It's a wonderful resource. One of the suggestions made by several of its contributing authors is for the primary caregiver of a person with dementia to create a "backup plan." Caregiving is the hardest work you'll ever do. Nothing is more taxing. You're bound to find yourself feeling unwell now and then. Even caregivers are allowed to be sick. Your backup plan may include these six things:

1. A complete medical history of your loved one: past medical issues, health conditions, surgeries, known allergies, the works!

---

1. See "Why We're Here" at https://www.thecaregiverspace.org/about/.

2. An updated medication list, with prescribing physician information, the pharmacy name and address, dosages, and times.

3. Backup caregivers' contact information: names, phone numbers, etc. Also, include any senior living communities that may be a good fit for your family member should that prove necessary.

4. Physician contact information and what condition your loved one see them for. (No one has just one physician these days, especially not someone with dementia.)

5. Medicare and insurance information, health insurance card, prescription card, etc.

6. Miscellaneous health-related documents, such as durable power of attorney, a living will, a DNR order, etc.

Don't forget to let several people other than yourself know where this information is kept. If you have an attorney, it may be a good idea to give him or her a copy. Your congregation's office may also be a place to store a copy.

Just having a backup plan—knowing you are not alone—can go a long way toward alleviating caregiver burnout. How do you know if you need a break? Burnout feels like a candle that ran out of a wick—it doesn't have what it needs to continue to provide light. Burnout can occur when you don't get the help you need personally, as you devote all of your time and energy to helping someone else. It can also happen when you try to do more than you're able to, emotionally, physically, or financially. Every rope can become frayed.

Your health and well-being matter just as much as the person you're caring for. It's important to know the signs and symptoms of caregiver burnout so you can get the help you need when you need it most. Believe me, if you are coping with feelings of frustration and stress, you are not alone. While it may seem difficult, taking a break from caring may be the best way to avoid:

- Passing on our sickness to the person we're caring for

- Feeling inadequate with the quality of care we're providing
- Worsening our own sickness or prolonging it further
- Saying something we might regret

Our congregation has a group of men who have trained themselves to provide support for those in need. I watched them care for a man who was unable to provide for even his most basic needs for months (they took turns being with him on a daily basis). Today, they regularly schedule short visits with people in order to give their caregivers a break. Sometimes even the shortest respite is enough to refresh a caregiver.

Still, it may be hard to leave your loved one in someone else's care, even if only for a few hours. When my father was in his final illness, my mother organized "Breakfasts with Bob" and had friends of his come over for a breakfast she'd fix. She'd have them eat together while she stayed in another room. It gave her a break of sorts, even though she herself wouldn't leave. She was always afraid "something would happen."

The Mayo Clinic website lists types of respite care that may be considered:

> • In-home respite. Health care aides come to your home to spend time with your loved one or give nursing services or both.
> • Adult care centers and programs. There are centers [some are in churches] that give day care for older adults. Some also care for young children. The two groups might spend time together.
> • Short-term nursing homes. Some assisted living homes, memory care homes and nursing homes accept people who need care for short stays while caregivers are away. [Hospice can also provide short-term respite care.][2]

Mayo even suggests that caregivers who work outside the home may think about taking a leave from a job for a time if it can be afforded. "Employees covered under the federal Family and

---

2. Mayo Clinic Staff, "Caregiver Stress," under "Respite Care."

Medical Leave Act may be able to take up to 12 weeks of unpaid leave a year to care for relatives. Ask your human resources office about choices for unpaid leave."[3]

If you need a break from caregiving to tend to your own emotional and physical well-being, and if you are unable to find family or friends or others to provide the kind of support you need, there is a national Eldercare Locator that may work. Provided by the US Administration on Aging, it connects older Americans and their caregivers with trustworthy local support resources.[4] The website mentions services such as meals; transportation; sitter services; and information about VA benefits, legal assistance, Medicare and Medicaid programs, and elder abuse or neglect.

LIVE-IN HELP

On World Communion Sunday 2023 I found myself in St. James Episcopal Church in Florence, Italy, a parish organized in the 1860s for the many American expatriates living there at that time. Its beautiful Gothic Revival building was completed in the early 1900s, with much of the funding coming from patrons such as Edward Francis Searles and J Pierpont Morgan.

A multicultural community, St. James welcomes worshippers from all over the world. I had great fun trying to guess the nationality of those I met. In particular, I spoke with a woman from England who told me all about her twenty years in Italy and about her husband, a retired academic. She pointed him out a few rows ahead of me and said he was the white-haired one sitting with his *badante*. I nodded as though I understood what she meant.

Later, while talking with the rector, I was told that *badante* meant "caregiver." Italy is still a very traditional culture with a strong bias toward families taking care of their own. Yet, with more and more families needing two incomes, leaving *Nonno* or

---

3. Mayo Clinic Staff, "Caregiver Stress," under "Working Outside the Home."

4. See https://eldercare.acl.gov/Public/Index.aspx.

Nonna home alone is problematic. One solution is a more or less live-in caregiver. A *badante*.

According to Carla Facchini, a sociologist at the University of Milan, "the rise of the 'live-in careworker' ('badante') model has been strongly facilitated by . . . the process of globalization that has occurred in the last two decades."[5] Italy's aging population and the world's unprecedented emigration have combined to produce the badante phenomenon as "a way of maintaining a household-centered model even in the occurrence of a downsizing of the care work carried out by the families."

In other words, as more and more Italians become "non-self-sufficient" due to age and/or dementia, and as fewer families are able to provide the needed care, there are immigrant workers available to do just that. Facchini concludes, "The development of this model of care apparently is a winning strategy for all stakeholders: for the older person and their families, for the badante, for the countries involved."[6] In some instances Italy's National Health System defrays the cost of the *badante*.

This arrangement is not without its critics. A report on Yale-Global Online from 2017 calls it "Modern Servitude."

> As Europe confronts the challenges of an aging population, workers from relatively poor countries relocate to wealthier communities to provide care. "Badante" is an Italian term for caregiver that also refers to foreign women, especially the Romanians who leave home and family to work long hours for low pay in Italy.[7]

It is my understanding that most of these caregivers have no medical training or certification of any kind. They don't provide that kind of support. They are there to help, to provide companionship, and to generally assist with the activities of daily living. I asked my new English friend what the *badante* did for her husband. She said, "Everything—helps him get up in the morning,

5. Facchini, "Caring," under "The 'Live-in Careworker' Model," para. 7.

6. Facchini, "Caring," under "Positive Factors and Critical Aspects of the Immigrant Live-in Careworker Model," para. 1.

7. Besliu, "Modern Servitude," abstract.

get dressed, get 'out and about,' ready for bed at night—whatever is needed."

We can all be *badanti*! Friends, neighbors, and church members can help provide respite within limits, perhaps in rotation. And they should! But as a person's dementia advances, the debate over formal live-in caregivers versus an assisted living facility versus a nursing home gains traction.

In the United States, some insurance companies—including Medicare—provide respite care (in a health care facility) in order to give a caregiver a break. As health care costs continue to rise, it may actually be less expensive to have around-the-clock live-in caretakers than it would be to place your loved one in a nursing home or memory care unit. However, regardless of which option is ultimately chosen, the needs of both the person with dementia and the primary caregiver of that person are both vitally important. The plea "do not forsake me" is still heard.

Chapter Ten

Live-In Care versus Assisted Living versus Nursing Home

Carry each other's burdens, and in this way you will fulfill the law of Christ.

—GAL 6:2

THERE IS A PROGRESSION that families go though in providing dementia care. It usually starts with simply keeping a closer eye on Mom or Dad (or whomever). Then it advances to something quasi-structured: taking them out to eat or having them over for dinner on a regular basis. If there is more than one child, conversations about them and their care begin taking place. A neighbor or pastor may call one of the children to express concern.

Eventually, someone in the family (usually the child living nearest) starts taking a much closer interest in them and their affairs. Appointments and medications are monitored. Trips to the doctor are no longer unaccompanied. Are the bills being paid? Who cuts the grass? Who maintains the home? The car keys are eventually taken away (with great difficulty)! Caregiving in earnest has now begun. This kind of caring vigilance may last for months or even years. It can work well too! Most dementias are slow developing, and with planning and help, people can safely live independently for a long time.

Then it happens. Almost always the issue of live-in caregiving help versus assisted living versus nursing home is unavoidably brought on by a crises of some sort: there is a fall down a flight of stairs and a broken arm. Or a UTI develops, or a bedsore is discovered. Someone walks away from a pot of marinara sauce on a hot burner on the stove and doesn't notice the smoke or even hear the smoke alarm. Something must be done. The time for denial is over.

When I was a pastor in Knoxville, one of our older members (at the time, she was ninety years old) moved into an assisted living facility. Upon my first visit to her there, she told me how much she hated it: everybody was old! Everyone wants to stay home. Home is familiar. It's where our stuff is. Our memories are associated with it, and our lives are inextricably entangled with where we live, especially if we have been there a long time. Staying at home is often "better" (whatever that means) for those with dementia, so considering an assisted living community or a nursing home for a person for whom you are caring is a daunting task.

First of all, no guilt! By the time the illness has progressed this far, the primary caregiver has done yeoman duty. But enough is enough. Pastors and priests can go a long way toward alleviating the guilt a caregiver feels when he or she has reached this point by reassuring them that they are struggling with the same issues tens of thousands of others are struggling with. (Figures are hard to come by, but there may be as many as three million people in dementia care facilities in 2024.) Sometimes the best way to love someone is to let go: let go of them in your home or in your 24/7 care or from being under your watchful eye.

LIVE-IN CARE

The pros and cons of live-in care are obvious. Your loved one can remain in the comfort of their own home, where everything around them is familiar. You can have a say in who provides care for your loved one. Care can be tailored to your loved one's individual needs. You will have some flexibility with scheduling and hours of care. (Keep in mind that the cost of in-home care will vary depending on the number of hours of care required.)

On the other hand, it can be difficult to find qualified, reliable caregivers. You may need to provide transportation for the caregiver to get to and from your loved one's home. The cost of in-home care may fluctuate if the needs that are addressed increase or change, making it difficult to budget. How comfortable are you with a stranger in the house? How comfortable will your loved one be with a stranger in the house? I know a family that had to draw up a "contract" with "Mother" in order to keep her from firing her caregivers. The contract included a provision that only her son could fire someone. She had to be reminded of this fairly often!

One of our members was fortunate enough to find a "companion" to help her live independently. (Actually, her family found her new "friend," but it was presented as her own idea.) This friend cooked for her, did a little light housekeeping, drove her to the store and to the beauty parlor, and was someone to talk to. Before leaving for the night, the companion fixed a simple dinner and made sure the house was secure. Our member was able to tuck herself in bed and wore a medical alert button on a lanyard around her neck. Next day, the companion would arrive and it would start over. It was a happy and pleasant arrangement that lasted years. It was sort of a *badante* model of caring support.

The bottom line is that deciding on live-in or nursing home care depends on an accurate assessment of the kind and type of care your loved one needs, as well as what the primary caregiver needs. And where such care is needed. If you work, either in an office or at home, but are otherwise available to provide care in the evenings and at night, either in your own home or in theirs, a part-time or even full-time live-in caregiver may be the right call. Such a person could help out during the day while you take care of the night. And there may be help to pay for such care. For instance, Medicare may pay for up to thirty-five hours a week of home health care for people certified as "homebound."

The biggest caveat to in-home care is the first "con" listed above: qualified and reliable. Just who can be a formal caregiver?

How do you find one? Where do you start? There can be real panic when contemplating this. Internet sites such as Care, SeniorAdvisor, A Place for Mom, etc., are places to start. Another avenue is the Alzheimer's Association chapter in your area. A comprehensive site on all things dementia-related is Alzheimers.gov. The section entitled "Tips for Caregivers and Families of People with Dementia" is especially insightful.[1]

NURSING HOME/MEMORY CARE

If you have been taking care of Mom or Dad at home (yours or theirs), and their dementia can no longer be considered "early" stage, the time for moving them into an assisted living community may be past. By definition, an assisted living facility is "a residence for people who require help with some of the routines of daily living."[2] Residents of assisted living communities are free to come and go. Many of them still drive. They are able to dress themselves and make it to the dining hall on their own. Such places are not equipped to deal with wandering or sundowners. What you may need is a nursing home or memory care home. Even many assisted living communities now have a memory care "wing" or "unit," so you may have more options than you realize.

A dementia care facility or memory care center is a type of nursing home designed with dementia care in mind. The AARP says that memory care is "a form of residential long-term care that provides intensive, specialized care for people with memory issues."[3] The pros and cons of a dementia care facility are similar to those of live-in care, with several significant differences. Pros include around-the-clock care and supervision, which can be a relief for caregivers who need a break or who live far away. These facilities are also supposed to have staff trained in dealing with

---

1. Alzheimer's, "Tips for Caregivers."
2. Investopedia Team, "Assisted Living," para. 1.
3. Crouch, "Memory Care," para. 2.

dementia-related behaviors. Also, facilities offer additional services such as social activities and therapies that may be of benefit.

On the downside, dementia care facilities can be expensive. In some cases very expensive. The *New York Times* ran a depressing series of articles entitled "Dying Broke" in 2023 that exposed just how shockingly expensive dementia care is.[4] Not every resident adjusts well to living in a communal setting. Unfortunately, there is also the potential for abuse or neglect in any facility, so it's important to do your research and visit several before making a decision. (Do not make the mistake of assuming that abuse or neglect cannot happen with live-in care either.)

Not all facilities are created equal. You really will have to do your homework. I have visited people in a dementia care home where all the residents were placed in one large room every day for hours at a time. There was little care in evidence, and no enrichment for the residents at all. By the same token, I have been to other facilities and seen wonderfully kind staff tending residents with compassion and grace. If your pastor or rabbi regularly makes rounds at area nursing homes, he or she could be a valuable resource for you.

In-home care and dementia care facilities are both viable options for those struggling with memory loss. While it is important to consider the needs of your loved one when making this decision, it is also important to consider your own needs. A therapist friend of mine once told me, "Do the math!" If caregiving is liable to disable or sicken you, then it is time for a change. If you are removed from the equation, who will care for your loved one? Ultimately, whichever option you choose should be what will provide them—and you—with the most comfort and help.

4. *New York Times*, "Dying Broke."

Chapter Eleven

Philosophy of Care

Finally, all of you, be like-minded, be sympathetic, love one
another, be compassionate and humble.

−I Pet 3:8

While visiting an "Alzheimer's village" in Monza, Italy, I saw
interactions between residents with dementia and caregivers that
I have rarely seen in the United States. The four *r*'s of dementia
care—reassure, reconsider, redirect, and relax—were seemingly
effortlessly employed.[1] It changed my perspective on the kinds of
interactions that ought to take place with people with dementia,
especially with those in the early and middle stages of the disease.
All too often I have seen and heard dementia patients referred to
like infants: "baby," "sugar," "sweetie," "honey," etc. Terms like this
are meant for endearment, especially in the South, but they come
off as disrespectful. They infantilize the patient. The patients' real
names are rarely used. Their personhood is violated enough by
disease. They do not need thoughtless caregiving adding to it.

MONTESSORI FOR DEMENTIA CARE

While it may be possible to find a wonderful at-home caregiver
who has no training or certification for the position, who ends

1. Most, "Caring for Loved One," para. 4.

up checking all the boxes you look for, certified caregivers should always be the case when considering a dementia or memory care center. They are supposed to be professionals. Always ask which approach the facility uses in caring for their residents. As you tour the place, as you look around for yourself, see if you find evidence of the care they say they use. One philosophy of care you may look for is Montessori.

Yes, that Montessori. Developed by an Italian physician (Maria Montessori) in the early 1900s, the Montessori educational method evolved out of observations that children in "confined" situations needed more stimulation in their environment than was being provided. Today, the Association Montessori Internationale and the American Montessori Society cite as essential to their method such things as mixed-age classrooms, student choice of activities (within a limited range of options), uninterrupted blocks of work time, and a "discovery" model of instruction.

Hands-on activities are emphasized. For instance, students may use sandpaper cutouts to learn letters. Or they learn math concepts by using beads. Each of the five senses is brought into play as much as possible. Peer-to-peer involvement is encouraged. Activity, communication, exploration, and repetition characterize a Montessori classroom, which makes the Montessori method an ideal framework, not only for children but for dementia care too. Dementia patients in confined situations need stimulation in their environment too.

In 2014, the Association Montessori Internationale invited dementia experts from around the world to form the first Montessori Advisory Group for the application of the Montessori approach for persons living with dementia. The key takeaway from their work is that while Montessori for adults with dementia may be simple and uncomplicated, it is not childish or simplistic. Among other things, the advisory group recommended that caregivers make use of a person's remaining capabilities, recognizing that even a person with dementia has the ability to improve some skills with practice, that all people—even those with dementia—need to be as independent as possible, and that social roles should be encouraged and strengthened.

IL PAESE RITROVATO

Il Paese Ritrovato is the Alzheimer's village I mentioned above. It was created and organized "to feel like a small town where guests can live a normal life, feeling at home but also receive proper treatment."[2] I was impressed with how little it looked like a medical facility. Nor did it have that "institutional" feeling about it.

It consists of eight apartment buildings, each with eight single rooms plus a bathroom for each. The total number of "guests" is sixty-four. Each of the eight rooms opened onto a community living room, a small kitchen, and what was referred to as an "assisted bathroom" large enough for a person to have someone nearby to provide help. There was a flat-screen television in the living room. The modular furniture was simple and easy to move, and stout enough to get in and out of without too much effort. Each eight-room unit had the feel of a new college dormitory.

The rest of the complex—about five acres in all—included several public squares, brick-paved streets, gardens, a theater, a beauty salon/barber shop, a church, and a sort of a general store with a cafe on one side. There was also a *gelateria*. I saw a dozen or more outdoor seating areas with benches, tables and chairs, arbors, awnings, and canopies. There were game tables and puzzles, all outside. There were two walking paths and a fruit tree orchard. All in all, it was a lovely place to visit.

Although my Italian is pretty limited, and the English of some of the staff I spoke with was similarly challenged, I heard the term "guest" used repeatedly. Not "resident" or "client" and certainly not "patient." Those on the staff were dressed in a way that was indistinguishable from the guests, except for a small name tag. No one wore lab coats or nursing uniforms or scrubs. The equality

---

2. CFS Italia, "Paese Ritrovato," para. 1.

of appearance was obvious, at least to one used to the hierarchical uniforms of US facilities.

One of the outdoor features I saw was a table set up in front of the general store with various household items on it. The first time I strolled past it I took a photograph. There was a stove-top espresso maker, an ancient cast iron skillet, a wireless brass lamp, a dusty rolling pin, and some pots and pans. I asked about them and was told that the guests like to touch and examine the items. They pick them up and look intently at them. Run their hands over them. Sometimes, I was told, an item is taken back to a room. In the mornings, the staff gathers them up and puts them back on the table. Every week or so the items are exchanged for others. It was this table that made me think that Montessori principles influenced the way Il Paese Ritrovato operates. Il Paese Ritrovato, by the way, translates as something like "the remembered community."

During my conversations with a physician on staff, I was told that every effort is make to encourage the guests to be outside: to walk outside, to sit with others, to stroll in the gardens, to visit the shops, to take in the fresh air, to listen to the birds, and to just enjoy life. She said the private rooms are small by design so the guests cannot easily hide away in them. Televisions are in common areas, and meals are served in each apartment's common dining room. I was told by several different staff members that no one is alone here. Independent, yes, as much as possible, but not alone. Socialization is all important.

On one visit there I was invited to attend a performance of "the drama club." About twenty-five of us gathered in the theater, which was large enough to host everyone in the village. There was a stage across one end, with padded folding chairs along the side walls and back. The woman in charge of the club visits Il Paese Ritrovato twice a week. She began by calling us to order and assigning parts. Since I would not do well with a speaking part, I was told I would be a tree. There were four or five of us trees, each holding branches cut from the orchard. When she pointed at us, we would wave the branches and make sounds like the blowing wind.

Other guests were given scripts to read from, there was a brief consultation about "blocking," and off we went, acting out scenes from favorite movies. I can't swear to it, but I think one of the scenes was from Casablanca. One of the men wore a fedora, another sat at a piano with a white tux jacket on (way too large for him), while a woman wearing a long string of pearls was appropriately distressed over whatever it was that was being said. And all the time the trees were waving and blowing in the background.

As I left after my final visit, I asked the medical director if their way of providing care was working for the guests. She said she and the staff were keeping as detailed a record as they could, and that they were convinced that the guests experienced fewer "incidents" and needed less medication than in other facilities. She added that quality of life is hard to measure but that that was their goal: to provide their guests with the best life as long as possible.

I learned there are other efforts being made in relation to dementia care in Italy. For instance, there are multiuse facilities that combine nursing homes with nursery schools. In Piacenza, these kinds of interactions take place:

> On one side of a glass wall, three toddlers in a nursery school flattened play dough with plastic rolling pins. On the other, three old women in a nursing home tapped the pane to get their attention.
>
> "Let's say hi to the nonni," the children's teacher said before leading them through a door that connected the two rooms.
>
> The children stopped to play with the magnifying glass of a delighted 89-year-old woman who had been using it to read obituaries. Then the toddlers, all 2 years old, took an elevator upstairs, where nursing home residents waited to read them picture books in a small library.[3]

While in Italy I heard of other such arrangements, such as intergenerational camps and housing that intentionally places the elderly side by side with young families.

---

3. Horowitz, "Double Whammy," paras. 1–3.

Italy was the first country in the world to adopt a nationwide dementia care plan—approved in 2014—and begin to provide funds for it. Admittedly, it hasn't gotten very far, but it's a start. Its intention is the "support of patients and families throughout the pathways of care."[4] So far there are 534 Centers for Cognitive Disorders and Dementias, and each one is charged with fulfilling the national plan's goal. One wonders if a national plan of some sort would make a difference in the US.

4. Di Fiandra et al., "Italian Dementia National Plan," abstract.

Chapter Twelve

Visitation

Carry each other's burdens, and in this way you will fulfill the law of Christ.

–GAL 6:2

I STILL REMEMBER HOW incensed I became when a woman I visited on a regular basis told me that no one else ever visited her, not even her children or grandchildren. "And they live right here in town." A few days later I had a phone call from her son who had been to see her, and he was upset that no one from the church ever visited his mother. "After all she's done for your church over the years." That's when it first dawned on me that providing pastoral care for someone is not without unexpected challenges. Eventually he and I realized that in her mind no one ever did visit her and that she was unable to remember even when someone did visit.

Sometimes you just can't win! But if you and/or your congregation systematically make the effort to care for those you know who have dementia, you will go a long way toward evening the odds. By "systematically," I mean regular visitation. Keep a logbook or some other sort of record of your visits. If there is a family member or close friend of the person you are visiting, let them know of your contact with their loved one. You don't have to do this every time but often enough so they know you are visiting. The care you provide in person to a family member with dementia may open doors for pastoral care to other members of the family. It has to be comforting to them to know that someone they care about is also being seen by others who care.

VISITING IN A CARE FACILITY

Earlier in this book, I said I was interested in related questions: How does one care for a person with dementia before any sort of institutional intervention occurs, and afterwards as well? And, how does one care for that person's caregiver before any sort of institutional intervention occurs, and afterwards as well? Much of what has preceded this chapter has dealt with providing care to the one with dementia prior to moving (or being moved) into a nursing home or memory care center. Now it is time to focus specifically on how to navigate such facilities.

First of all, are you even allowed to be there? Do not assume! Some facilities have a policy of not allowing visitors for the first several weeks a person is there. Repeated occurrences of COVID, RSV, the flu, etc., have caused many types of care facilities to be more cautious in allowing indiscriminate visitation. HIPPA concerns may also prevent you from visiting. A quick phone call to check visitation policies can save a lot of trouble. While on the phone, ask when is a good time to visit. Mornings are busy times in care facilities. Lunch time or the early afternoon is almost always preferred. Call the family too. It may be rare, but sometimes a primary caregiver does not want a facility to allow any visitors at all. Remember, you are visiting at the convenience of the resident and the family and the staff.

Also, do not be surprised if you are asked to wear a mask. However, this can be problematic: it may protect someone from infection, but at the same time it can interfere with recognition. All of us rely on the faces we see to process "the feelings, intentions, desires, and mental states" of those we interact with.[1] People with dementia find this excruciatingly difficult. Add a mask that covers

---

1. Kynast et al., "Mindreading from the Eyes," abstract, para. 1.

most of a person's face, and communication with that person becomes nearly impossible.

There are two steps you may take to overcome this. First, do not visit anyone in a care facility if there is even the slightest chance you have been exposed to an illness. Second, if you do go and are asked to wear a mask, ask if you can take it off when visiting a person in private. Or, barring that, ask if you can take it off momentarily in order to reassure the person who you are, then put it back on in that person's presence. Remember to clearly state who you are, your name, and your connection to that person. Call them by name. If the mask is too distracting or intimidating, you may have to simply try later. The last thing you want to do is add to a person's agitation or confusion.

Once you are at the facility, check in at the receptionist's desk. Introduce yourself, and name the person you are there to see. A visitor's log is usually available to sign in, with space for the time you arrived, the time you left, and whom you visit. (This written record keeps all of us honest when we are asked—or challenged—about our visitation habits.)

I generally spend time with the person I am there to see wherever I find him. If he is in his room, we visit there. (Always knock before entering.) If she is in a dining hall or the library, that's where we'll spend time together. Occasionally I will come across someone walking the halls or enjoying the outdoors. If they are walking, I will walk. If they are outside, I will stay outside with them. A visit to someone with dementia is all about that person. If at all possible, I try to avoid imposing my agenda on them. Interrupting their day may upset them, something I try to avoid.

TALKING

Talking to a person with dementia in a nursing home or memory care center is much like talking to them in their own home. The same suggestions apply: introduce yourself, and ask if he or she would like you to visit them. If so, it is up to you to carry the conversation. Keep in mind the advice Alzheimer's San Diego gives:

"Don't reason, don't argue, don't confront, don't remind them they forgot, don't question recent memory, don't take it personally."[2] And don't forget to pause every once on a while so they can respond. Give them time to speak. Your silence alongside them is not a bad way to communicate.

I find it helpful to think of conversation as a way into their world, not a way to somehow inform them of my world. What I mean by this is that I will talk about their life as best I can. Their hometown, their family, their work, their church. I do this until I make a connection, however small it might be. If I never connect, it is still time well spent. Maybe my role can be to remind them of their own life events. Or not!

One afternoon I sat with one of our members who is struggling with dementia. He is a wonderful man, still at home, with a supportive family and many friends. Speech has become more difficult for him: when he attempts to talk, he mostly sputters out something we have to guess at. On this day as we chatted I rehearsed his career—without asking what he remembered. I said something like "How gratifying it must have been for you to be a pediatrician. A baby doctor. You had all kinds of options for what kind of doctor to be, and you chose to take care of children."

As usual, he had been mostly silent as we talked, but after I finished the above he blurted out, "They were so much easier than adults." I was astonished at how clearly he said this. Then he added, "I could always make a child laugh. Then I could talk to them about their problem." He had obviously been following my conversation as I spoke and responded accordingly. We never know how much or how little is being perceived, hence our need to be respectful and to assume they are able to understand us even if they cannot respond.

Suzanne Finnamore wrote a guest essay for the New York Times entitled "Dementia Is a Place Where My Mother Lives. It Is Not Who She Is." She finds it helpful to think of her mother living in a land called Dementia, and reminds us that "living in

2. Summarized from Alzheimer's San Diego, "Do's and Don'ts"; emphasis added.

Dementia isn't the defining chapter of her life."[3] This is why I insist on using a person's real name. We use it during every other chapter of a person's life; there is no reason not to if they have dementia. Our names have meaning. They have been with us our entire lives. Finnamore also writes, "There is dignity in Dementia if we say there is."[4] How we talk with dementia patients, how we treat them, how we care for them will go a long way toward maintaining their dignity. If they can't do it themselves, we can do it for them.

Finally, do not forget the person who has been the primary caregiver. We all tend to the follow the patient. If we visited him or her at home, we will visit him or her in a memory care center. But we cannot forget to visit the primary caregiver, whose life has now been upended—once again—by dementia.

---

3. Finnamore, "Dementia Is a Place," para. 22.
4. Finnamore, "Dementia Is a Place," para. 23.

Chapter Thirteen

Learning to Live Again

The Lord appeared to us in the past, saying: "I have loved you
with an everlasting love; I have drawn you with loving-kindness."

—JER 31:3

THINK ABOUT IT: FOR many months now a primary caregiver's life
has been almost completely consumed with caregiving! Morning,
noon, night, repeat. Morning, noon, night, repeat. Doctor appointments, home health visits, people coming and going at all hours
providing a variety of services, friends calling, pastors stopping by,
unexpected trips to the hospital, and precious little "alone" time.
(Alone? What's that?) How to fit in a trip to the grocery store? Are
the bills being paid? Does the house need a good dusting? Worry
upon worry, stressor upon stressor. The carousel keeps on spin-
ning. And then it stops. Your loved one is in a nursing home. Now
what?

It is vitally important that those who regularly visit a person
with dementia not neglect that person's primary caregiver once a
medical facility of some kind has come into the picture. According
to a 2017 study published in *The Gerontologist*, "three overarching
themes" emerged from interviews with former caregivers: sleep
disturbances, changes in health status, and difficulty learning to
live again.[1] The understated conclusion of this study is that "there

1. Corey and McCurry, "When Caregiving Ends," abstract, under

74

may be long-term effects of caregiving on health that persist well beyond the first year post-caregiving."[2]

A Place for Mom seconds the above by listing the specific challenges dementia poses to caregivers: "While caregiving may be necessary and rewarding, it can also lead to health risks for family caregivers."[3] The reason is obvious. Dementia care is "high intensity," meaning that it takes significantly more time and energy than other types of care. The social isolation and financial hardships are stressful. And dementia caregiving is long term: lasting, on average, five years or more. All of which can leave a caregiver with anxiety, depression, and loneliness. We know that chronic stress is a killer. Mortality rates bear this out: 18 percent of healthy spouse caregivers actually die before their partner with dementia.[4]

LIFE AFTER CAREGIVING

My mother spent four years caring for my father during his final illness, but he did not have dementia, which meant she was able to leave him alone for an hour or so at a time. She was able to go to church, or to the store, or to make a quick visit to see a friend. She did not have to learn to live again the way she would have had to if he had had a different illness. Caregivers of those with dementia are not so fortunate. A faith community can be a literal lifeline for them.

In the same way that those with dementia need to be intentionally, regularly visited when in their home and in a medical facility, the primary caregiver needs to be visited too. When both are at home, it is be possible to see and support caregiver and care receiver at the same time. But once a nursing home is in play, separate visits will inevitably be necessary. This is how it should be. Visiting a person who has spent months or even years caring for

---

"Results."

2. Corey and McCurry, "When Caregiving Ends," abstract, under "Implications."

3. Samuels, "Major Health Risks," para. 1.

4. Samuels, "Major Health Risks," under "Increased Mortality Rate."

a loved one in his or her home helps to normalize being at home alone. You can visit with both of them at the nursing home, of course, if the caregiver is there. But that is best if it occurs organically, as an unintended consequence of regular pastoral visits to the nursing home, and you just happen to be there when the caregiver is too. Seeing both parties at the same time is no substitute for seeing each one individually.

Normalizing being alone—learning to live again—means different things to different people. But at least one of the things it means to practically everyone who has been a primary caregiver is picking up those things of importance that have been placed "on the back burner" while caregiving. Health concerns, family and social relationships, work-related issues, hobbies and other outside interests, and financial matters can all be attended to in ways not previously possible. All of which may be overwhelming!

Remember, too, that caregiving has its rewards. It isn't just the burden of care that has eased up but the joy and sense of purpose it brings as well. If a person has been caring for another for a long time, his or her identity may be wrapped up in providing care. Having the loved one placed in a home may signal failure on his or her part, or the identity as a person is called into question if one is no longer the primary caregiver. Normalizing may mean rediscovering who you are as a person.

POST-CAREGIVER STRESS DISORDER

Since the COVID pandemic, it is fashionable for some clinicians to talk about PCSD—post-caregiver stress disorder. Of course, it existed long before COVID! Sometimes called "caregiver PTSD" (post-traumatic stress disorder), this condition is characterized by physical, mental, and emotional exhaustion.[5]

Caregiving has a substantial impact on the caregiver's health. Note: it isn't that it *may* have an impact; it does. For instance,

---

5. Ingber, "Caregiver Stress Syndrome," para. 1.

- Eleven percent of caregivers state that their role as caregiver has caused their physical health to decline.

- Forty-five percent of caregivers reported chronic conditions, including heart attacks, heart disease, cancer, diabetes, and arthritis while caregiving or afterwards.

- Caregivers have a 23-percent higher level of stress hormones and 15-percent lower level of antibody responses than non-caregivers.

- Ten percent of primary caregivers report that they are under physical stress from the demands of assisting their loved one physically. (Think of a 150-pound woman lugging around a 250-pound man!)

- Women who spend nine or more hours a week caring for a spouse increased their risk of heart disease by 100 percent.

- Seventy-two percent of caregivers report that they have not gone to the doctor as often as they should have.

- Fifty-eight percent of caregivers state that their eating habits are worse than before they assumed this role.

- Caregivers between the ages of sixty-six and ninety-six have a 63-percent higher mortality rate than non-caregivers of the same age.[6]

A study published by the *International Journal of Environmental Research and Public Health* entitled "Risk and Protective Factors for PTSD in Caregivers of Adult Patients with Severe Medical Illnesses" identified the following sociodemographic and socioeconomic characteristics of those likely to suffer caregiver PTSD: being a female caregiver (especially a younger female); having a lower income (fewer options for help?); and having a lower level of education.[7]

When it came to familial relationships, the same study found that having a closer relationship with the patient (being spouse or

6. Family Caregiver Alliance, "Caregiver Health."

7. Carmassi et al., "Risk and Protective Factors," sect. 3.1., para. 2.

parent) was a factor related to PTSD symptoms. Being a spouse is a higher risk; being a parent is a lower one. Also, predictably, having a more enmeshed and chaotic family system places one at higher risk for PTSD, as does experiencing more days of patient hospitalization and higher levels of persistent patient's pain.[8] Does this mean the more time spent at a loved one's bedside, the more likely you are to develop caregiver PTSD? I imagine that is the case, especially if they were in pain, but more context would be helpful here!

ALL IS NOT LOST

One of the points I've made throughout this book is the importance of pastoral care for both the one with dementia and the one providing their care. The study above indicates that social status, familial relationships, support, and the ability to cope positively are factors associated with lower PTSD symptoms. Continuing to work, having a higher educational level, being the child of the patient (instead of a spouse or a friend), and a high level of social support all decrease PTSD symptoms.

All is not lost. Once your loved one is in a medical facility, while you will visit often—even daily—you will have more time on your hands than you have had in years. Learning to live again is something that will take time. It can be painful too. "Moving past loss and finding a new sense of purpose after years of caregiving is a gradual, up-and-down process."[9] However, make no mistake: there is life after caregiving.

Amy Goyer writes, "Like many family caregivers, my role as caregiver for my parents had become an enormous part of my identity. It gave me a deep sense of purpose and, for so many years, was behind all of my personal and work-life decisions."[10] It is precisely here that a faith community can be most helpful. The

---

8. Carmassi et al., "Risk and Protective Factors," sect. 3.1., para. 3.

9. Wynn, "How to Reclaim Life," deck.

10. Goyer, "Life after Caregiving," para. 4.

church is heir to the promise "I have come that they may have life, and have it to the full" (John 10:10). There is something healing in simply being part of something larger than yourself. There is love and grace and forgiveness when participating in worship and service with others. Being part of a faith community is a reminder that the final word on who we are—and on those we care for—is not ours but God's.

Chapter Fourteen

For All the Saints

Share with the saints who are in need. Practice hospitality.

−ROM 12:13

A FAVORITE OBSERVATION OF mine about the early church as portrayed in the New Testament is that the word "saint" never appears. At least, not in any Greek text. I know what you are thinking: What about Saint Matthew? Or Saint Mark? Or Saint Luke? Or Saint John? Those are sometimes included in the titles of the four Gospels. They were added to the text centuries after they were written, partly in order to tell them apart, and partly to honor the traditional author of each one. The word "saint" does not appear in the New Testament. Instead, what we have is the plural, "saints." No one is a saint. There are only saints. We are saints only when we are with each other.

What we do for each other is epitomized in one of the psalms: "As iron sharpens iron, so one person sharpens another" (Ps 27:17). Most scholars interpret this to refer to the influence we have on each other, some sort of refinement of character. I like to think that making each other sharper means we make each other better, stronger, more caring, more loving. It fits with what I've seen in relation to dementia care: people helping other people care for people who cannot care for themselves results in better care than is possible alone. Iron sharpens iron. The result is "group" sainthood.

I have served five different congregations over the course of more than forty years. For most of my ministry I have been responsible for pastoral care. I have learned much about life and faith from the saints I've known, especially from those dealing with dementia. With dementia comes a lot of pain, not to mention grief, along with joy and just plain human goodness. But, a dementia-aware congregation is able to deal with the bad as well as the good. Do not be naive. Here are three cautionary tales.

SCAMMED

In West Virginia I knew a woman—a widow—living alone, who claimed to be a descendant of the "Richards Wild Irish Rose" wine family. (I looked this up one time and decided she was pulling my leg.) She was always dressed to the nines, always smiling. White hair, powdered face. She was never without a cane, which she mostly used to point. Unfortunately, in her case I learned how easy it is to scam a person with early dementia, something every dementia caregiver needs to take seriously.

She had a house full of antiques, and when it came time for her to "break up housekeeping" and enter an assisted living facility, an antique dealer "from across the river" who had befriended her offered to sell her most valuable pieces on consignment. Item after item was taken from her home by people she did not know. She was completely befuddled by it. There was no record of what had been taken. She said people just put things in boxes and took them. When she asked the dealer for a list of items intended for sale, it was never clear if the list that was finally produced (months later) was complete or not. Those of us who had been in her home thought not! We were fairly certain she was never paid for what was taken. She mourned her antiques until she could not remember them anymore, and could not understand how "those nice people" could do that.

A FALL AT HOME

The first person I knew to be diagnosed with frontotemporal dementia was a man from Knoxville, well educated with an expansive vocabulary. He used to say that he "liked ten-cent words and five-cent cigars." He also said that he "never used a five-cent word when a ten-cent word would do." A defense attorney by profession, he was a spellbinding storyteller by avocation. (His church school class still reminisces about his stories!) He retired when he realized he was having trouble finding the right words to argue his cases. We, too, noticed his struggles with self-expression. By the time he died, he was barely able to speak and could no longer read. He spent hours sitting silently in a chair.

His illness brought with it increasingly poor balance. The home he and his wife lived in—on a lake with a spectacular view—was not a house someone with dementia could easily navigate. But modifications were made as best as they could. Safety bars were put near the toilet and in the shower, etc. There were conversations about moving to another home, and they nearly bought into a retirement community but ultimately decided against it. He wanted to be in his own home. His wife supported him in this. We all did. One evening he fell on the stairs. He died after a short stay in an ICU.

WHERE DID HE GO?

One of the elders of our church in Chattanooga, a retired assistant manager of a municipal golf course, divorced and living alone, began stopping by the church more frequently than had been his habit. He had been a member for years, and had served on our property committee, so we didn't mind his visits. But he began to stay for hours. Sometimes he would talk to one of our staff members, usually about the building or grounds. Sometimes he would hardly speak at all but would quietly hum to himself. Or he would just sit and stare. All in all, it was unnerving.

We thought he was just lonely. At loose ends. He was a nice man, a kindly man, very faithful to our church. When we closed because of the COVID pandemic, we lost touch with him. After we began meeting again, he was noticeably absent. When we telephoned him, there was never an answer. Eventually one of our members and I drove to his house to see if we could find him. We did. He was there, along with a woman who said she was his daughter, but who knows? The house was in shambles. He greeted us warmly but without recognition. We went back later only to find the house empty. A few weeks after that, we received a note saying that he was being taken care of in her home in another state. We tried to contact her after that, to no avail. We never heard from him again.

Being scammed, falling down, or just plain disappearing are among the more unfortunate risks associated with dementia. Need I say that they are reasons to have a community of faith to help dementia caregivers? In hindsight, I am convinced that the outcomes for the woman whose antiques were taken and for the man who disappeared would have been different had we been more alert to what they were dealing with. Dementia is particularly perilous for people who live alone. As for the man who fell down the stairs, he was where he wanted to be, and all things considered, was functioning pretty well when he died. Isn't that how we'd all like to go?

COMMUNITY EFFORTS

I know of three organized attempts by congregations to address dementia's growing crises and provide respite for caregivers. The first is called Let's Sing From Memory, which meets twice a month from 10 to 11:30 a.m. at a Chattanooga Methodist church. It's open for anyone to attend and is similar to a program popular in the UK. Basically, it's a sing-along for both those with dementia and their caregivers. Singing stimulates a part of the brain that isn't often tapped into.

The second program, held in dozens of congregations throughout the South, is called Abide Respite Ministry. It is designed to provide friendship for its participants as well as a break for their caregivers. Meeting Tuesdays and Thursdays each week, from 10 a.m. to 2 p.m. Abide combines music and pet therapy, chair exercise, arts and crafts, intergenerational activities, and service projects for those who come.

Third, Greenville, South Carolina, is home to Side by Side, a volunteer-driven, community-outreach ministry of John Knox Presbyterian Church. Similar to Abide, Side by Side meets twice a week, 10 a.m. to 1:45 p.m., and seeks to provide a break for individuals living with memory loss and their caregivers. Everyone needs a breather! Enriching conversations, lively games, craft activities, lunch, music, exercise, service projects, and worship are all part of the program.

FOR ALL THE SAINTS

On October 31, 2023, my wife and I and a couple of friends watched Italian children moving up and down the streets of Morbegno dressed as witches and ghosts, asking shop owners and passersby for treats. It was Halloween! They were having such a good time, it was hard not to smile. After dinner, we asked our hosts if anything was planned for us for the next day. No, we were told: they were going to visit the graves of their parents, but maybe the day after that we could go somewhere nice. The next day, of course, was November 1—All Saints Day. Italians have a deep-seated belief that there is a powerful spiritual bond between those who are living and those who have died. It's a connection that is never really broken. And so it is with those who live with and suffer with and ultimately die with dementia. They are simply the saints who now rest from their labors. In time, we, too, shall follow.

Chapter Fifteen

Where to Go for Help

Each of you should look not only to your own interests, but also to the interests of others.

—PHIL 2:4

THIS MORNING ON MY iPhone's news feed are the following sensational headlines: "Medicine Stopped in 1980s Linked to Rare Alzheimer's Case," taken from BBC News; "Scientists Find Evidence Alzheimer's Can Be Transmissible," Gizmodo (health); a related headline, "Alzheimer's Passes between Two People for the First Time in Recorded History," *Irish Star*; "Owning a Pet May Lower Risk of Dementia for Adults 50 and Older," *People*; and "Vital Early Signs of Dementia Can Be Spotted While Supermarket Shopping," BuckinghamshireLive. Clearly, the world has awakened to the problem of dementia. Information is out there. But the question now becomes, where to find reliable help?

Even though we know not everything on the internet is worth paying attention to, an internet search is where more and more people begin a hunt for information on most things. So that's where we'll begin.

INFORMATION ABOUT ALZHEIMER'S DISEASE ON THE INTERNET

I heard a professor once say that a Google search is not research. But it is if it gets you to right place! I suggest you start digging for information on dementia—and especially on Alzheimer's disease—by going to the Alzheimer's Association's website.[1] The home page includes basic statistics about the disease, the prevalence of the disease in each state, comments on caregivers, and updates on treatments. The "help & support" and "local resources" links are invaluable. Look for a local branch of the Alzheimer's Association in your community. There is also a European Alzheimer's Association[2] and one for the United Kingdom.[3]

There are a host of other websites with accurate, helpful information: the National Institute on Aging,[4] the Centers for Disease Control,[5] the World Health Organization,[6] Alzheimer's Disease International,[7] and an official website of the United States government[8] are just a few of them. The Vanderbilt Memory and Alzheimer's Center is a source of information on current scientific work on Alzheimer's,[9] as is the Center for Alzheimer's Disease Research at Brown University.[10]

Other reputable sources of information and support include the Mayo Clinic,[11] the Cleveland Clinic,[12] Johns Hopkins

---

1. www.alz.org.
2. www.alzheimer-europe.org.
3. www.alzheimers.org.uk.
4. www.nia.nih.gov.
5. www.cdc.gov.
6. www.who.int.
7. www.alzint.org.
8. www.alzheimers.gov.
9. www.vumc.org.
10. www.alz.carney.brown.edu.
11. www.mayoclinic.org.
12. www.clevelandclinic.org.

University,[13] Stanford University,[14] and Houston Methodist Hospital's Nantz National Alzheimer's Center.[15]

INFORMATION ABOUT DEMENTIA CAREGIVING ON THE INTERNET

Caregiving sites are a mixed bag. For one thing, some of them are nonprofit, some of them aren't. Some of them are aligned with a particular clinic or medical practice or nursing home chain and are designed to "drive" business toward them. It is important to read up on the sponsor of the sites you peruse.

For instance, the first response to a search I made on Google for "dementia caregiving" was "Dementia Care," sponsored by Thrive Senior Living of Lookout Mountain, Georgia. The second response was entitled "Compassionate Caregivers," sponsored by BrightStar Care, a home health company with "franchising" as one of its offerings. "Dementia & Alzheimer's Care" came up third. It was the title of a website run by Storypoint, a memory care and assisted living facility in Chattanooga. Still, I found good information on all of these sites and ignored the chat boxes that popped up wanting to send me more information about their facilities.

Eventually I got to nonprofit information on caregiving on a page by the Alzheimer's Association. Alzheimers.gov also came up, as did the AARP, and Houston Methodist. All of the organizations listed above, those under the "Information about Alzheimer's Disease on the Internet" heading, also have pages on caring for someone with dementia.[16]

---

13. www.johnshopkinsmedicine.org.

14. www.stanfordhealthcare.org.

15. www.houstonmethodist.org.

16. You can find helpful articles at www.alzheimersreadingroom.com, www.dementia.org, www.dementiacarestrategies.com, www.thecaregiverspace.org, and www.caregiver.org.

OTHER SOURCES OF INFORMATION ON THE INTERNET

A Place for Mom is a ubiquitous website for a privately held, for-profit senior care referral service headquartered in New York.[17] Its services are free to families, and it receives funding from the senior living communities and home care providers on its platform. In other words, it markets the senior housing communities and home care providers it refers to families that use it. (It also owns and runs SeniorAdvisor.com, a consumer ratings and review site for senior care providers across the US and Canada, which sounds sort of like the fox rating the henhouse.) Still, I have found stories and articles on A Place for Mom that I have cited in this book. Just be careful where you look and what you sign up for. Brookdale Senior Living, Genesis Healthcare, Life Care Centers of America, Atria Senior Living, Elmcroft Senior Living, and MorningStar Senior Living are just a few of the health care "chains" that dominate dementia care facilities. They may all provide help and support, but as I said earlier, be careful what you sign up for.

INSTITUTIONS AND AGENCIES WORKING ON DEMENTIA CARE

I have already mentioned the "big guns" of dementia research: Cleveland, Mayo, Vanderbilt, etc. Agencies such as the National Institute on Aging, the National Council on Aging, the Administration on Aging, Centers for Disease Control and Prevention, and nationwide organizations such as the Dementia Society of America are reputable sources of information and guidance.

The Nantz National Alzheimer Center at Houston Methodist Hospital in Houston, Texas, deserves special mention. Founded in 2011 by sportscaster Jim Nantz, it has become a world-renowned research and referral center, treating thousands of patients each year. Its stated goals are "to prevent Alzheimer's disease, slow memory loss progression, and improve the quality of life for every

17. www.aplaceformom.com.

patient."[18] On a personal note, one of our church members has been to the Nantz Center, and his wife couldn't be more positive about the experience. While her husband was undergoing cognitive testing, she spent an hour with a physician who spoke with her about dementia, her husband's experiences with it, and her own thoughts and feeling about it.

Locally, in East Tennessee, we have not only a chapter of the Alzheimer's Association, with an office in Knoxville, but also Alzheimer's Tennessee. Both serve our region of the country, providing information, support, and the vision of a future world without dementia. A great way to get involved with others working to end dementia is by participating in a Walk to End Alzheimer's.

BOOKS ON DEMENTIA CAREGIVING

For those of you who still like the feel of a book in your hands as you read, the list of volumes on dementia in all its facets is increasing daily. My efforts are primers compared to some of them. I always recommend *The 36-Hour Day*, by Nancy L. Mace and Peter V. Rabuns. First published in 1981, there have now been seven editions. A review by Alex Raftakis for Arbor Terrace Naperville (one of those assisted living communities that produces insightful information even as it uses that information to drive business for itself) calls it "the archetypal how-to manual on how to manage and solve problems caused by dementia."[19] *Learning to Speak Alzheimer's* by Joanne Koenig Coste emphasizes communication between caregivers and patients and encourages us to relate to those with dementia in their own reality. Pauline Boss coined the term "ambiguous loss" to refer to types of loss "without closure." She explores this concept as it relates to dementia in *Loving Someone Who Has Dementia: How to Find Hope While Coping with Stress and Grief*.

18. See homepage of https://www.houstonmethodist.org/neurology/centers-and-programs/nantz-national-alzheimer-center/.

19. Raftakis, "Book Review," para. 2.

There are many others, of course. Most poignant are those firsthand accounts of the disease, such as *While I Still Can . . .*, by Rick Phelps and Gary Joseph Leblanc. Rick was fifty-seven years old when he was diagnosed with early onset Alzheimer's disease. The Memory People social networking site on Facebook that he started is still running. For insight into what is it like to have Alzheimer's, this book is a must-read. *Into the Storm: Journeys with Alzheimer's*, edited by Collin Tong, is a twenty-three-writer anthology of caregivers from all walks of life sharing their stories of caregiving.

THE BLESSING OF THIS BOOK

As I have worked on this book, and on its predecessor,[20] I have become more and more impressed with the resilience, fortitude, and grace dementia caregivers demonstrate by what they do. It is no accident that the "care" we have been talking about is referred to as "given." While I am sure some care is given grudgingly, what I have read about, heard about, and seen for myself has been freely and lovingly given. It's been a tremendous gift poured forth, knowing it can never be repaid. I am convinced that in some unfathomable way, when people give of themselves to someone else, and that giving calls forth every ounce of strength and love that they have, and yet they still do it, they are walking a sacred path.

My prayer is that this book will be a blessing to others as even as I have been blessed by those caregivers who have crossed my path.

> For I am convinced that neither death nor life, neither angels nor demons, neither the present nor the future, nor any powers, neither height nor depth, nor anything else in all creation, will be able to separate us from the love of God that is in Christ Jesus our Lord. (Rom 8:38–39)

---

20. Rader, *Do Not Cast Me Away.*

Concluding Thoughts

ONE AFTERNOON, AS I was contemplating how to end this book, I was told of a woman whose husband constantly asked her where they were going or what they were going to do. She hit upon the idea of putting a note in his pocket every morning with the day's activities on it. Now, for the most part, instead of asking her again and again, he takes the note out of his pocket, looks at it, then puts it back in his pocket. Then he takes it out again . . . Caregivers learn to adapt to dementia, each in their own way. There is no way to end this book, because I keep learning about living with dementia. I just decided it is time to stop writing for a while.

JAIL TIME

My son (the public defender) recently told me a disturbing story. A man with dementia got into a car that was not his own. Unfortunately, the keys were in it. He managed to start it up and drove off. Inevitably, he had a fender bender. He was arrested and charged with auto theft.

The man had no identification and could not tell the arresting officers his name or where he lived, so he was placed in the county jail. I suppose they thought someone would come looking for him, but no one did. The sheriff's department never found out who he was. This was in one of Tennessee's poorer counties. There were no resources to work with this man to find out who he was, where he lived, or if he had family somewhere. He quietly sat in his jail cell, never caused a problem, and was there for months.

Jails receive reimbursement from the state based on the daily census. The truth of the matter is that there was no incentive to help this man get out of jail, few resources to work with him if someone did want to help him get out, and a strong financial incentive to keep him in jail.

I thought this was surely an isolated case until I saw an article in the *New York Times* written by Katie Engelhart about Federal Medical Center Devens, a prison in Massachusetts for prisoners who require medical care.[1] It includes a Memory Disorder Unit that currently houses two dozen men with dementia. Furthermore, it is estimated that there are thousands of other persons with dementia incarcerated in American prisons. So much for my isolated case!

Our ethical dilemma is stark: How can we punish a prisoner for his crimes when he no longer remembers them? Engelhart says it's a complicated matter:

> Within the philosophical literature on cognitive impairment, there is a debate about whether a person with advanced dementia is even the same person as he was before. If he cannot be considered the same person, then the men of the M.D.U. are, in an important sense, being punished for someone else's crime.[2]

Can we hope for dementia-friendly prisons?

DEMENTIA-FRIENDLY CONGREGATIONS

Faith communities of all types are developing resources to create dementia-friendly congregations. The Discipleship Ministries of the United Methodist Church has a checklist for churches to consider:

1. Are all areas of the church clutter-free, well lighted, and mapped out or marked where they lead? Are there adequate storage places available for unused items? Is there a process

1. Engelhart, "I've Reported on Dementia."
2. Engelhart, "I've Reported on Dementia," para. 44.

for checking to make sure items are put away when they are not in use in public areas?

2. Are classrooms free of complicated and misleading stimuli? Have you minimized background noise (radio, TV, computer, overhead speakers)?

3. What are the expectations of caregivers when church members visit their family member who has dementia? Are caregivers' needs being met with support groups? Are respite programs available? What strategies have been developed to deal with behavioral difficulties of those with dementia?

4. Have you simplified tasks and directions so that everyone, including people with dementia, can follow them?

5. In what ways is the church engaging people with dementia to prevent boredom, depression, and agitation while they are present? In what ways are church programs helping members with dementia experience service to others, purpose, joy, and hope? How can the skills and abilities of those with dementia be best used during their time at church to give them a sense of being normal?

6. What activities does the church offer that help to maintain the current cognitive function and spirituality of members with dementia? What new activities could a church offer, such as art therapy or dementia-oriented worship, which could be a family event?

7. What role can the church play in preserving the history and relationship of people with dementia with other members of the church? (For example, recording their memories before they are lost.) What opportunities exist to help those with dementia continue to express who they have been in life? Do activity designs allow people to be remembered for who they are, and not for their illness?

8. What is a church's "Plan B" for ministering to members with dementia and caregivers when they are no longer able to continue to participate in church activities? How will the church

continue to minister effectively to, for, and with members when they become homebound or move to a skilled medical center?

9. Have you completed educational programs and training for leaders about dementia? Have you taken into consideration the needs of church members with dementia and their caregivers?

10. Has a careful study of the building and grounds been undertaken? Have the following areas been checked? Restrooms, kitchen, storage areas, etc.[3]

THE COMING TSUNAMI

The world's aging population is sometimes called "the silver tsunami." I'm afraid that a tsunami is coming, and it won't be easy to deal with. Perhaps you've had similar thoughts as you've read this book. Four converging phenomena may spell disaster for many of the institutions we have enjoyed in our lifetimes if we don't begin to address them now. They are: the increasing number of people with dementia, the concomitant number of people who will be forced into dementia caregiving (most of them during their prime employment years), the rising costs of geriatric health care, and the decline of geriatricians.

At the risk of being pedantic, let me add some data. The number of those with dementia will rise to approximately twelve million by 2050. By that date the number of dementia caregivers will be somewhere above twenty million. The annual cost for providing dementia health care will be right at $1 trillion dollars. Currently, in 2024, there are only 7,300 geriatricians in the United States. It is estimated that we will need 30,000 of them by 2050.[4]

---

3. Discipleship Ministries, "Dementia-Friendly Church," under "Dementia-Friendly Church Checklist."

4. Rowe, "US Eldercare Workforce."

Can we complete a fundamental shift in how we fund and provide health care for those we love? And not just for those we love or those who are elderly or those who have dementia but for everyone? Our congregations can go a long way toward making this happen, but it will take activism, as well as commitment, on our part.

A POEM ON DEMENTIA

A few years ago the Alzheimer's Society published a poem, "When My Grandad Had Dementia," written by a thirteen-year-old for World Poetry Day, March 21, 2018. It pushes all the right buttons. I included parts of a poem in this book's introduction. I find it fitting to close with one. God bless you and your loved ones.

"When My Grandad Had Dementia," by Katelan Carter

It was a hard time in our lives
When my Grandad had dementia.
He found things hard and would suffer,
So my Nan was like a carer.

He used to mix me and my sister up,
When my Grandad had dementia.
Bonnie was his favorite pup,
And she used to nap with him on the sofa.

His steps were slow, stiff and heavy,
When my Grandad had dementia.
But then one night we got a call,
About his terrible fall.

Mum went to see him at hospital,
When my Grandad had dementia.
I tried to see the light of the tunnel,
Playing on the swings at the park.

One day at school snow started to fall,

Do Not Forsake Me

When my Grandad had dementia.
In my heart I knew it was a sign,
I wondered whether everything was fine.

After school I got told the news,
And instantly my heart broke and bruised.
He wasn't coming home,
Instead to heaven he went.

When my Grandad died with dementia.

Bibliography

Ali, N., et al. "Risk Assessment of Wandering Behavior in Mild Dementia." *International Journal of Geriatric Psychiatry* (2015). https://doi.org/10.1002/gps.4336.

Alzheimer's. "Tips for Caregivers and Families of People With Dementia." Alzheimer's, n.d. https://www.alzheimers.gov/life-with-dementia/tips-caregivers.

Alzheimer's Association. "Late-Stage Caregiving." Alzheimer's Association, n.d. https://www.alz.org/help-support/caregiving/stages-behaviors/late-stage.

———. "Sundowning." Alzheimer's Association, last updated Jan. 2023. https://www.alz.org/media/documents/alzheimers-dementia-sundowning-ts.pdf.

Alzheimer's Caregivers Network. "A Caregiver's Guide to Sundown Syndrome: How to Recognize and Manage Symptoms." Alzheimer's Caregivers Network, Jan. 3, 2023. https://alzheimerscaregivers.org/2023/01/03/7-steps-to-choosing-professional-alzheimers-care-providers/.

Alzheimer's San Diego. "Communication Strategies." Alzheimer's San Diego, Sept. 2019. https://www.alzsd.org/wp-content/uploads/2021/09/COMMUNICATION-Communication-Strategies-Updated-3.3.21.pdf.

———. "Do's and Don'ts of Communication and Dementia." Alzheimer's San Diego, n.d. https://www.alzsd.org/dos-and-donts-of-compassionate-communication-dementia/.

ASPE. "A Profile of Older Adults with Dementia and Their Caregivers Issue Brief." ASPE, Sept. 2018; published Jan. 23, 2019. https://aspe.hhs.gov/reports/profile-older-adults-dementia-their-caregivers-issue-brief-0.

Besliu, Raluca. "Modern Servitude: Romanian Badante Care for Elders in Italy." YaleGlobal Online, Jan. 3, 2017. https://archive-yaleglobal.yale.edu/content/modern-servitude-romanian-badante-care-elders-italy.

Boss, Pauline. *Loving Someone Who Has Dementia: How to Find Hope While Coping with Stress and Grief.* San Francisco: Jossey-Bass, 2011.

Brodaty, Henry, and Marika Donkin. "Family Caregivers of People with Dementia." National Library of Medicine, 2009. From *Dialogues in Clinical Neuroscience* 11 (2009) 217–28. https://pubmed.ncbi.nlm.nih.gov/19585957/.

Carmassi, Claudia, et al. "Risk and Protective Factors for PTSD in Caregivers of Adult Patients with Severe Medical Illnesses: A Systematic Review." *International Journal of Environmental Research and Public Health* 17 (2020) 5888. https://doi.org/10.3390/ijerph17165888.

CDC. "Caregiving for a Person with Alzheimer's Disease or a Related Dementia." CDC, last reviewed June 30, 2023. https://www.cdc.gov/aging/caregiving/alzheimer.htm.

CFS Italia. "Il Paese Ritrovato." CFS Italia, n.d. https://www.cfsitalia.com/en/projects/il-paese-ritrovato/.

Churchill Retirement Living. "New Top 10 'Grandfluencers' List Shows That Age Really Is Just a Number!" Churchill Retirement Living, n.d. https://www.churchillretirement.co.uk/news/retirement-lifestyle-news/top-10-grandfluencers/.

Ciccone, Isabella. "Caregivers [*sic*] Perceived Reciprocity Reduces Behavioral Symptoms in Patients with Alzheimer Disease." NeurologyLive, July 16, 2023. https://www.neurologylive.com/view/caregivers-perceived-reciprocity-reduces-behavioral-symptoms-in-patients-with-alzheimer-disease.

Clinebell, Howard. *Basic Types of Pastoral Care & Counseling: Resources for the Ministry of Healing & Growth.* Updated and revised by Bridget Clare McKeever. 3rd ed. Nashville: Abingdon, 2011.

Corey, Kristin L., and Mary K. McCurry. "When Caregiving Ends: The Experiences of Former Family Caregivers of People with Dementia." *Gerontologist* 58 (2018) e87–e96. https://doi.org/10.1093/geront/gnw205.

Coste, Joanne Koenig. *Learning to Speak Alzheimer's: A Groundbreaking Approach for Everyone Dealing with the Disease.* Boston: Houghton Mifflin, 2003.

Cottle, Michelle. "You Shouldn't Have to Take Care of Your Aging Parents on Your Own." *New York Times*, Sept. 6, 2023. https://www.nytimes.com/2023/09/06/opinion/seniors-home-care-aging.html.

Crouch, Michelle. "Memory Care: Specialized Support for People with Alzheimer's or Dementia." AARP, Dec. 6, 2021; updated Mar. 26, 2024. https://www.aarp.org/caregiving/basics/info-2019/memory-care-alzheimers-dementia.html.

Dementia UK. "Tips for Communicating with a Person with Dementia." Dementia UK, Oct. 2003. https://www.dementiauk.org/information-and-support/living-with-dementia/tips-for-communication/.

Di Fiandra, Teresa, et al. "The Italian Dementia National Plan." ResearchGate, Jan. 2017. https://www.researchgate.net/publication/291838206_The_Italian_dementia_national_plan.

Discipleship Ministries. "The Dementia-Friendly Church." Discipleship Ministries, Sept. 29, 2015. https://www.umcdiscipleship.org/resources/the-dementia-friendly-church.

Engelhart, Katie. "I've Reported on Dementia for Years, and One Image of a Prisoner Keeps Haunting Me." *New York Times*, Aug. 11, 2023. https://www.nytimes.com/2023/08/11/opinion/dementia-prisons.html.

Everman, Lynda, et al., eds. *Dementia-Friendly Worship: A Multifaith Handbook for Chaplains, Clergy, and Faith Communities*. London: Kingsley, 2019.

Facchini, Carla. "Caring for Non-Self-Sufficient Older People in Italy: From a Familistic System to the Immigrant Live-in Careworker Model." CAPP, n.d. https://capp.iscsp.ulisboa.pt/images/CPP/V6N2/5_V6_N2.pdf.

Family Caregiver Alliance. "Caregiver Health," 2006. https://www.caregiver.org/resource/caregiver-health/.

Finnamore, Susan. "Dementia Is a Place Where My Mother Lives. It Is Not Who She Is." *New York Times*, May 8, 2022. https://www.nytimes.com/2022/05/08/opinion/dementia-elder-care.html.

Firth, Shannon. "Preventing Gun Violence in Patients with Dementia." MedPage Today, Sept. 23, 2021. https://www.medpagetoday.com/geriatrics/dementia/94663.

Gobel, Brandon. "Laundry Pods Killing Dementia Patients." AARP, June 26, 2017. https://www.aarp.org/health/healthy-living/info-2017/laundry-pods-killing-dementia-patients-fd.html.

Goyer, Amy. "Life after Caregiving: The Unexpected Beginning." AARP, Oct. 20, 2020. https://www.aarp.org/caregiving/life-balance/info-2020/finding-purpose-after-caregiving-ends.html.

Grey, Heather. "Alzheimer's, Caregiving, and Managing Frustration." Healthline, June 15, 2023. https://www.healthline.com/health/alzheimers/alzheimers-caregivers-managing-frustration.

Hamilton, Jon. "Big Financial Costs Are Part of Alzheimer's Toll on Families." NPR, Mar. 30, 2016. From *Morning Edition*. https://www.npr.org/sections/health-shots/2016/03/30/472295791/big-financial-costs-are-part-of-alzheimers-toll-on-families.

Hauerwas, Stanley, et al., eds. *Growing Old in Christ*. Grand Rapids: Eerdmans, 2003.

Horowitz, Jason. "The Double Whammy Making Italy the West's Fastest-Shrinking Nation." *New York Times*, Jan 30, 2023. https://www.nytimes.com/2023/01/30/world/europe/italy-birthrate.html.

Ibrahim, Shannon. "Demi Moore Speaks Out on Ex-Husband Bruce Willis' Dementia Battle: 'Let Go of Who They've Been.'" *New York Post*, Jan. 31, 2024. https://nypost.com/2024/01/31/entertainment/demi-moore-speaks-out-on-ex-bruce-willis-dementia-let-go-of-who-theyve-been/.

Ingber, Ron. "Caregiver Stress Syndrome." Caregiver, n.d. https://caregiver.com/articles/caregiver-stress-syndrome/.

Investopedia Team, The. "Assisted Living: What It Is, Paying for It, Options." Investopedia, last updated Jan. 17, 2022. https://www.investopedia.com/terms/a/assisted-living.asp.

Khachiyants, Nina, et al. "Sundown Syndrome in Persons with Dementia: An Update." *Psychiatry Investigation* 8 (2011) 275–87. https://doi.org/10.4306/pi.2011.8.4.275.

Kynast, Jana, et al. "Mindreading from the Eyes Declines with Aging—Evidence from 1,603 Subjects." *Frontiers in Aging Neuroscience* 12 (2020) 550416. https://doi.org/10.3389/FNAGI.2020.550416.

Lindeberg, Sophia, et al. "Conversations in Dementia with Lewy Bodies: Resources and Barriers in Communication." *International Journal of Language & Communication Disorders* (Dec. 2022). https://doi.org/10.1111/1460-6984.12799.

Linthicum, Dorothy, and Janice Hicks. *Redeeming Dementia: Spirituality, Theology, and Science.* New York: Church, 2018.

Mace, Nancy L., and Peter V. Rabins. *The 36-Hour Day: A Family Guide to Caring for Persons with Alzheimer's Disease, Related Dementing Illnesses, and Memory Loss in Later Life.* Rev. ed. Baltimore: Johns Hopkins University Press, 1991.

Mannen, Sara. "Thinking Botox with Barth: Toward a Theology of Beauty with Aging." Center for Barth Studies, Feb. 13, 2024. https://barthcenter. substack.com/p/thinking-botox-with-barth?utm_source=publication-search.

Mayo Clinic Staff. "Caregiver Stress: Tips for Taking Care of Yourself." Mayo Clinic, n.d. https://www.mayoclinic.org/healthy-lifestyle/stress-management/in-depth/caregiver-stress/art-20044784.

McFadden, Susan H., and John T. McFadden. *Aging Together: Dementia, Friendship, and Flourishing Communities.* Baltimore: Johns Hopkins University Press, 2011.

McKeever, Amy. "Why Evenings Can Be Harder on People with Dementia—and How to Cope." *National Geographic,* Mar. 2, 2023. https://www.nationalgeographic.com/science/article/sundowning-syndrome-symptoms-causes-treatments.

Mitchell, Jerry. "History: Emmy Winner Cicely Tyson Born." *Mississippi Clarion Ledger,* Dec. 19, 2017. https://www.clarionledger.com/story/news/local/journeytojustice/2017/12/19/week-civil-rights-history-december-18-through-24/964490001/.

Most, Doug. "Caring for a Loved One with Dementia? BU Neurologists' New Book Offers Guidance." Boston University, Sept. 21, 2021. From Andrew Budson and Maureen O'Connor, *Six Steps to Managing Alzheimer's Disease and Dementia: A Guide for Families* (New York: Oxford University Press, 2021). https://www.bu.edu/articles/2021/andrew-budson-and-maureen-oconnor-six-steps-to-managing-alzheimers-disease-and-dementia/.

Newmark, Amy, and Angela Timashenka Geiger. *Chicken Soup for the Soul: Living with Alzheimer's and Other Dementias.* Cos Cob, CT: CSS, 2014.

New York Times. "Dying Broke." *New York Times,* Nov.–Dec. 2023. https://www.nytimes.com/series/dying-broke.

———. "William Saroyan Is Dead at 72; Wrote 'The Time of Your Life.'" *New York Times,* May 19, 1981. https://www.nytimes.com/1981/05/19/obituaries/william-saroyan-is-dead-at-72-wrote-the-time-of-your-life.html.

Nussbaum, Martha C., and Saul Levmore. *Aging Thoughtfully: Conversations about Retirement, Romance, Wrinkles, and Regret.* New York: Oxford University Press, 2017.

Ollivier, Debra. "Edith Pearlman, PEN Award Winner, on Success Late In Life." *HuffPost,* Nov. 29, 2011; updated Jan. 29, 2012. https://www.huffpost.com/entry/edith-pearlman-pen-award_b_1117158.

Phelps, Rick, and Gary Joseph Leblanc. *While I Still Can . . . : One Man's Journey through Early Onset Alzheimer's Disease.* N.p.: Xlibris US, 2012.

Rader, Paul. *Do Not Cast Me Away: Dementia in the Congregation.* Eugene, OR: Wipf & Stock, 2020.

Raftakis, Alex. "Book Review: *The 36-Hour Day.*" Arbor Terrace Naperville, n.d. https://www.arborcompany.com/locations/illinois/naperville/blog/book-review-the-36-hour-day.

Rowan, Anthea. "The Dreadful Physical Symptoms of Dementia." *Psychology Today,* updated June 22, 2023. https://www.psychologytoday.com/us/blog/were-only-human/202304/the-dreadful-physical-symptoms-of-dementia.

Rowe, John W. "The US Eldercare Workforce Is Falling Further Behind." *Nature Aging* 1 (2021) 327–29. https://doi.org/10.1038/s43587-021-00057-z.

Samuels, Claire. "Dementia and Wandering: Causes, Prevention, and Tips You Should Know." Place for Mom, last updated Jan. 21, 2021. https://www.aplaceformom.com/caregiver-resources/articles/dementia-wandering-causes-prevention.

———. "Major Health Risks for Dementia Caregivers." Place for Mom, Dec. 11, 2023. https://www.aplaceformom.com/caregiver-resources/articles/health-risks-for-dementia-caregivers.

Shakespeare, William. *As You Like It.* Edited by Barbara Mowatet al. Folger Shakespeare Library, n.d. https://www.folger.edu/explore/shakespeares-works/as-you-like-it/read/.

Shulman, Elizabeth. *Finding Sanctuary in the Midst of Alzheimer's: A Spiritual Guide for Families Facing Dementia.* New York: Morgan James, 2021.

Span, Paula. "Caregiving's Hidden Benefits." *New York Times,* Oct. 12, 2011. https://archive.nytimes.com/newoldage.blogs.nytimes.com/2011/10/12/caregivings-hidden-benefits/.

Swaim, Emily. "Why Ageism Happens and How to Address It." Healthline, Mar. 30, 2022. https://www.healthline.com/health/ageism.

Taylor, David. "Monday Motivation: Five Inspirational Quotes by Feminist Betty Friedan." *Dan's Papers,* July 13, 2020. https://www.danspapers.com/2020/07/monday-motivation-betty-friedan/.

Tong, Collin, ed. Into the Storm: Journeys with Alzheimer's. N.p.: Book Publishers Network, 2014.

UNC School of Medicine. "Aging America: the Growing Need for Geriatricians." UNC School of Medicine, Aug. 17, 2023. https://www.med.unc.edu/medicine/news/aging-america-the-growing-need-for-geriatricians.

United Nations Department of Economic and Social Affairs. "Article 1—Purpose." United Nations Department of Economic and Social Affairs, n.d. https://social.desa.un.org/issues/disability/crpd/article-1-purpose.

Vanauken, Sheldon. *A Severe Mercy.* 2nd ed. San Francisco: Harper & Row, 1980.

Willimon, Will. *Aging: Growing Old in Church.* Edited by Jason Byasee. Pastoring for Life: Theological Wisdom for Ministering Well. Grand Rapids: Baker Academic, 2020.

Wynn, Paul. "How to Reclaim Life after Years of Caregiving." Brain&Life, Dec. 2017/Jan. 2018. https://www.brainandlife.org/articles/reclaiming-life-after-years-of-caregiving-is-a-gradual-up.

Yang, Hyun Duk, et al. "History of Alzheimer's Disease." National Library of Medicine, Dec. 2016. From *Dementia and Neurocognitive Disorders* 15 (2016) 115–21. https://www.ncbi.nlm.nih.gov/pmc/articles/PMC6428020.

www.ingramcontent.com/pod-product-compliance
Lightning Source LLC
Chambersburg PA
CBHW072206270326
41930CB00011B/2552